COLON CANCER ANSWERS

Understanding and Fighting Colon Cancer

Bruce A. Feinberg, D.O.

PRESIDENT/CHIEF EXECUTIVE OFFICER
GEORGIA CANCER SPECIALISTS

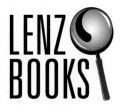

LENZ BOOKS

119 East Court Square, Suite 201
Decatur, Georgia 30030
www.lenzbooks.com

Lenz Books
119 East Court Sq.
Ste. 201
Decatur, GA 30030
www.lenzbooks.com

The authors, editor, and publisher have made every effort to provide accurate information. However, they are not responsible for errors, omissions, or for any outcomes related to the use of the contents of this book and take no responsibility for the use of the products described. Treatments and side effects described in this book may not be applicable to all patients; likewise, some patients may require a dose or experience a side effect that is not described herein. The reader should confer with his or her own physician regarding specific treatments and side effects. Drugs and medical devices are discussed that may have limited availability controlled by the Food and Drug Administration (FDA) for use only in a research study or clinical trial. The drug information presented has been derived from reference sources, recently published data, and pharmaceutical research data. Research, clinical practice, and government regulations often change the accepted standard in this field. When consideration is being given to use of any drug in the clinical setting, the healthcare provider or reader is responsible for determining FDA status of the drug, reading the package insert, reviewing prescribing information for the most up-to-date recommendations on dose, precautions, and contraindications, and determining the appropriate usage for the product. This is especially important in the case of drugs that are new or seldom used.

Colon Cancer Answers By Dr. Bruce Feinberg. ISBN 978-0-9798560-0-6

Production Credits
Executive Editor: Richard J. Lenz
Interior Illustrations: Imagineering
Composition: Matt Tinsley and Scott Sanders, Lenz, Decatur, Georgia
Cover Design: Scott Sanders, Lenz, Decatur, Georgia
Photo Research: Scott Sanders, Lenz, Decatur, Georgia
Printing and Binding: Asia Printing Co.
Cover Printing: Asia Printing Co.

Printed in Korea.

10 9 8 7 6 5 4 3 2 1

To Iris, Jon, Michael, Rachel, and Daniel,
Whose honesty keeps me humble;
Whose humor makes me laugh;
Whose love sustains me.

TABLE OF CONTENTS

TABLE OF CONTENTS (continued)

Preface

Approximately 150,000 Americans will be diagnosed with colon cancer this year, and a third will eventually lose their life to the disease. More than eighty percent of these cancer deaths would have been prevented had screening guidelines been followed. This is a preventable human tragedy.

Colon cancer is not discriminating. It affects men and women equally. It is not biased by race. Its only remarkable risk feature is age. Ninety percent of colon cancers develop in people over age fifty.

Surprisingly, despite the predictability of an age-related risk and the availability of an effective screening tool, colon cancer remains the second most common cause of cancer death in America. Why?

My own colonoscopy experience shed light onto the complex nature of the problem. I expressed indignation over the co-pay and deductible, since I was doing the "right thing" that would in the long run save my insurance company money. I was angered by the lost day of work. I obsessed over the bowel prep process with its required twenty-four hour clear liquid fast and double dose laxative. I agitated over the "what if there's a problem?" scenario.

My apprehension of the colonoscopy was ridiculous; however, my reactions and procrastination were all too common. At least fifty percent of at-risk, age-appropriate people in the United States undergo no colon cancer screening and possibly upwards of seventy percent fail to have a colonoscopy (the screening test gold standard). I rationalized my behavior by thinking my education and knowledge made my anticipation worse. All physicians have in their case records a patient who underwent a routine screening test that produced an unexpected and unfavorable outcome.

Could this same kind of thinking be the source of the anxieties that prevent millions of Americans from undergoing a colonoscopy? In my rational brain, I knew these routine health maintenance checks were a thousand times more likely to benefit me than disclose a problem for which there was no solution. But was this only because of my medical knowledge and experience? Was the problem with colonoscopy screening compliance due to financial reasons such as co-pay fees, deductibles and lost work? Or was the historical failure of Americans to undergo colon cancer screenings simply an anxious reaction to the indignity and sense of violation believed to accompany the experience? If people understood how devastating colon cancer can be and how totally preventable it is, would it change this irrational behavior?

I wrote this book with three goals: first, to provide a compassionate, understandable resource for the newly diagnosed. Second, to ease the fear, anxiety, and sense of helplessness of the loved ones and caregivers providing support to those with a diagnosis of colon cancer. And third, to dispel the myths of colon cancer. Myths that lead to irrational behaviors, which will result in millions of preventable colon cancer deaths this decade.

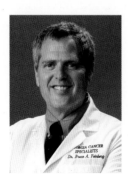

Dr. Bruce A. Feinberg

Why Cancer Answers?

I am a medical oncologist, a doctor who specializes in the treatment of cancer. After more than 20 years of patient care, I remain amazed by how little most people know about how their bodies work. Despite access to information via books, television, and the Internet, most people know much more about how their cars and appliances work than they do about their bodies. Even more surprising are people's responses when their bodies are broken. Most people will not hesitate to get two opinions about a funny noise in their car engine before forking over $1,000 to fix it. Ironically, these same people will go to the first doctor to whom they are referred and undergo a $10,000 potentially life-threatening procedure with no questions asked.

The car is a mechanical machine, whereas the body is an organic machine, albeit more complex, but not impossible to understand. I have observed that my patients who understand how their bodies normally work and how they are affected by disease feel more in control when they face serious illness. No disease is more serious than cancer, and none makes a patient feel less in control. My hope is that this book provides patients, their families, and their caregivers with the information that they need to gain control and to participate in critical decision making. Hopefully, as an active participant in their care, patients can improve their outcomes.

How To Use This Book

Colon Cancer Answers is an outgrowth of my consultations with newly diagnosed colorectal cancer patients. Over the years it became clear to me that simple illustrations were very effective in clarifying and reinforcing the explanations that I offered patients. My efforts to explain how the cancer began, how fast it was growing, whether had it spread, etc., were specifically enhanced with the illustrations. Despite the juvenile quality of my art, my patients often requested copies of the pencil drawings, as they helped them explain their situation to family and friends. One of my nurses suggested that I videotape a new patient discussion to improve my efficiency in the office, but I dismissed the notion as it seemed too impersonal. The suggestion did, however, trigger the thought that it would be wonderful if such a video or book were available for patients and families to have as a resource before and/or after the initial oncologic evaluation. I searched bookstores and web book retailers but could not find such a book. There seemed to be a real need for a colon cancer primer for patients. Colon Cancer Answers is designed to be such a primer. Each chapter builds on the information from the prior chapter. Illustrations accompany the narrative to reinforce and clarify the content. Keywords are in bold, indicating that they can be found in the glossary for future reference.

My favorite book in medical school was an anatomy text that was illustrated with layered transparencies. With the pages in place, the image was of a human body. When the first transparency was lifted, the skin was peeled away, exposing the underlying musculature. When the second transparency was lifted, the muscles were gone, and the skeleton was exposed. Subsequent transparencies exposed the organs, the circulation, and the nervous system. My hope is that this book peels away the confusion that confronts patients and their loved ones as each layer of the colon cancer problem is revealed.

To The Newly Diagnosed Patient

You have just been informed you have cancer. You are in shock. Your life is suddenly turned upside down. Don't panic! As ridiculous as it sounds, this is the best advice I can offer. To overcome the panic, you have to understand what is happening and what is going to happen to you. Your panic is rooted in the fear of the unknown and an irrational response to a situation of which you have no knowledge, no experience, and no control. Worse, you have only limited knowledge or indirect experience from cancer situations that are totally unrelated to the one that you are experiencing now. You are a newly diagnosed colon cancer patient, and your father's lung cancer and Aunt Ethel's leukemia are as different in behavior and outcome as are ice cream and artichokes.

In order not to panic and to gain control, you need to be educated about what has happened to your body and what should be anticipated. Unfortunately, seeking knowledge from well-intentioned friends and family or via the Internet is more likely to confuse than to comfort. Do not panic! With this book, the knowledge that you need to approach this disease with a positive attitude is provided.

Many types of cancer exist. With all cancers, cells in the body change and grow out of control. Usually, the multiplying cancer cells form a lump called a cancerous tumor. Cancerous tumors are also called malignant tumors. Sometimes malignant tumor cells can break away from the mass and travel through the bloodstream or lymphatic system to other parts of the body. This process is called metastasis. Not all tumors are cancerous. Those that are not are called benign. Cells from benign tumors do not spread to other parts of the body.

These statements seem straightforward enough and are probably adequate for the majority of people who have not encountered the most dreaded three words in the human language: You have cancer! However, when I am in the unfortunate situation of having to say these words to a new patient and his or her anxious loved ones, this explanation is woefully inadequate. Those involved need to know so much more. The questions are endless: Where did it come from? Why did it happen to me? When did it start? How far has it gone? How big is it? Has it spread? How can it be stopped, treated, and cured? For those who are actively battling colon cancer or who are supporting a spouse, child, parent, loved one, or friend who is suffering with colon cancer, this book is for you. This is the what, where, when, why, and how of colon cancer that hopefully will make sense of everything that you have heard, seen, been through, or are about to experience. In short, I hope to answer all of the questions about colon cancer that you may have—hence the title, *Colon Cancer Answers*.

Cancer is the most complex of human diseases. It begins with a step-by-step transformation of a single human cell. Because there are over 200 types of cells in the human body, over 200 types of cancer exist, each one distinct. How can I begin to explain the more than 200 most complex human diseases? First, I turn your attention to just one cancer, colon cancer. Then, I begin as the cancer does, with a single cell. I begin by examining the origin of a human cell and the progression to the 200 different types of cells that make up a complete body. You will learn about the cells that make up the colon and their normal structure and function. You will examine how their behavior changes as they transform into a cancerous or malignant state. I will discuss what causes this transformation as I explore cellular DNA, the genetic blueprint, or operating code that governs the cell's behavior. I will describe the natural history of colon cancer and how doctors use this knowledge to predict a cancer's course and plan its therapy. I will present the current strategies that medical science uses to both treat and prevent cancer. Finally, I hope to make sense of the gobbly gook of jargon, terms, and statistics that can either paralyze patients with fear or confuse them with false expectations.

Read this book cover to cover. Do not skip. Do not browse. Do not wander. I have specifically written this book to provide a step-by-step understanding of colon cancer. Like the layered transparencies of my medical school anatomy text that peeled away the external structure to reveal the inner workings, this book explains the transformation from the normal colon to colon cancer with all of its implications. The narrative is accompanied by illustrations that will assist you as you journey through the complicated world of medical jargon and statistics. Important key words and terms are in bold and can be found in the glossary. Take pauses to digest each chapter; read, go back, and reread if needed, but read methodically chapter by chapter. Use the illustrations found in each chapter to clarify and reinforce the narrative. This book is designed to be read in one evening and is going to eliminate hours, days, and weeks of emotional agony. Don't panic! Read this book!

Acknowledgements

This book would not be possible without the guidance, support, knowledge, wisdom, and friendship of Richard Lenz. Richard, more than anyone, helped me translate the passion with which I educate my patients into a vehicle with which to educate colon cancer patients and their loved ones everywhere.

I thank the skilled medical illustrators from Imagineering, who created the remarkable illustrations and helped set the narrative tone of the book. In particular I extend my appreciation to Jack Haley who guided the team of illustrators at Imagineering.

I would be remiss not to mention Deb Keen, my trusted assistant, whose help throughout the book's creation was invaluable.

To Fred Levine, my friend and gastroenterologist: not only did you make my colonoscopy completely forgettable, you also provided all the colonoscope images for this book. Thank you.

To Nishan Fernando my friend and colleague: I would not have considered this book publishable without your review of the scientific content; thank you. To Aileen O'Neill, Joanne Piratzky, and Charles (Buddy) Andrews, the best pathologists in Atlanta and a treasured community resource: my thanks for helping review the content. To my physician colleagues at Georgia Cancer Specialists: your compassionate and knowledgeable patient care is a continuous source of pride that has helped me grow as both a physician and a human being.

I am indebted to Scott Sanders who has the remarkable ability to translate my rambling, doodles, and scribbles into visual concepts that the illustrators could understand. To Matt, Michael, John, Pam, Ryan and the rest of the foos-ball crew at Lenz: thank you for helping to create *Colon Cancers Answers* and bring my vision to life.

To my loving family, especially my wife Iris, who put up with my insanity during my bursts of writing.

Finally, I need to express my gratitude to the many patients who have en-trusted their cancer care and their lives to my team of caregivers. I continue to be inspired by your courage and humbled by your grace. Physicians too often forget the gifts of knowledge and skill that allow them to help others during their time of need. I remember these gifts every day.

Making Sense of the Diagnosis

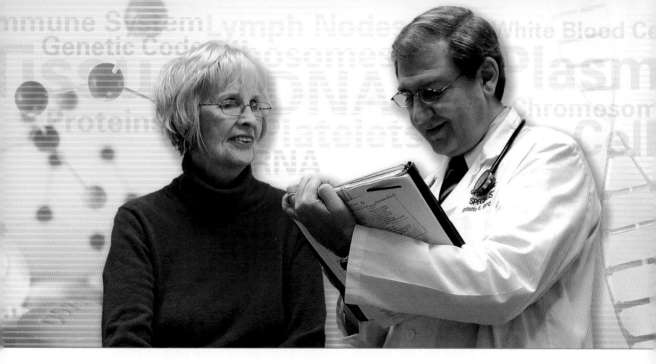

MEDICAL ONCOLOGISTS are physicians who take care of CANCER patients. Most medical oncologists, like me, restrict their practice to adult cancer patients. The most common adult cancers are those that originate in the body's ORGANS, such as the breast, colon, prostate, and lung. Rarely a week goes by that I do not see a new patient with a recently diagnosed cancer of the colon or rectum. Doris and Eric are such patients. Let me begin by introducing Doris.

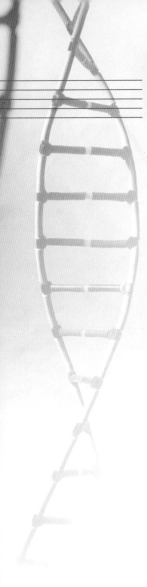

Introduction

Doris and her husband Sam were cruising the Panama Canal celebrating their 50th wedding anniversary when Doris had her first episode of rectal bleeding. It was easy for Doris to dismiss the episode rationalizing that the strain of travel, carrying heavy luggage, and eating rich foods were likely responsible. Doris also worried that she might have contracted a parasite while adventuring in one of the many ports of call. "Probably hemorrhoids," Sam said.

Doris had her second episode of bleeding a week later, after she and Sam had returned to their home in Atlanta. This episode was a bit heavier and scared her. Doris called her internist, Dr. Simon, who demanded she go to the emergency room, but as it was nearly dinnertime and she felt fine, she opted to wait and see him in the morning. Doris felt reassured by the facts: She experienced no pain, she had normal or what she had learned to accept as normal bowel movements every two to three days, and she had a normal COLONOSCOPY four years ago.

Dr. Simon had known Doris and Sam for 20 years. "Good people and good patients," he would tell his nurse. They were the model of good health and a healthy lifestyle. Sam still worked part-time, he played golf and tennis two or three times a week, and he could be found most nights and weekends in his woodshop in the converted garage. He also managed a daily one-hour walk with Doris, who like her husband, was always on the go with painting, pottery, watching the grandkids, and heading up the local knitting club. Dr. Simon liked to joke that he hoped he and his wife would be like Doris and Sam when they grew up. They were good patients because they watched their diets, exercised, and remained active, mentally and physically. They were also diligent with their annual physicals and health maintenance. Even with Sam's mild high blood pressure and Doris's osteoarthritis they were the poster children for healthy seniors.

When Dr. Simon first spoke to Doris on the phone, when she had called in reference to her bloody bowel movement, he considered hemorrhoids the source.

His exam suggested a more sinister source of bleeding. Doris's ABDOMEN was soft without tenderness, her bowel sounds were normal, but her rectal exam was not normal. Not only did Dr. Simon find red blood in the rectum but he also felt, at the tip of his finger, something hard. He hoped he was only feeling compacted STOOL and that the bleeding was related to internal hemorrhoids, but the possibility of cancer was inescapable. The intermittent bleeding, the absence of other gastrointestinal complaints, the normal ABDOMINAL EXAM, the absence of visible hemorrhoids, and the abnormal DIGITAL RECTAL EXAM all pointed toward a cancerous TUMOR involving the rectum.

After the exam was completed, Doris dressed and joined Sam in Dr. Simon's office. Dr. Simon was an open book, every emotion worn on his sleeve for all to see. This was a character trait that endeared him to his patients, but at this moment, his obvious concern for Doris's well being was raising Sam's blood pressure. "What's wrong?", Doris asked. Dr. Simon explained his findings and their implications. He made a list of all the possible explanations for her bleeding; a process physicians call the DIFFERENTIAL DIAGNOSIS. In this case, the differential diagnoses included cancer of the rectum at the top of the list.

Doris and Sam weren't children; they had many friends who had been through such medical moments. They were all business. "Tell us what to do next and it's done," Sam said. Dr. Simon explained that Doris needed to see Dr. Kanjavi or Dr. K. as he was often called. He was the GASTROINTESTINAL SPECIALIST who performed her last colonoscopy four years ago. Dr. Simon called Dr. K., explained his findings, and arranged for the office evaluation in the morning with the colonoscopy to be done the following day.

Dr. K. was very reassuring. He questioned Doris about her symptoms, examined her abdomen, and repeated the rectal exam. He then reviewed the preparation for the colonoscopy and the procedure itself. He explained that he would possibly need to perform a BIOPSY should he find an abnormality within the colon or rectum. Because a biopsy was likely, he would perform the colonoscopy in the hospital outpatient area rather than in his office. The word hospital seemed to echo in Doris's mind as its inclusion in the discussion suddenly raised the threat level of the problem. Dr. K. further explained that Doris would need to go by the hospital upon leaving his office for the preop testing and paperwork.

After the stop at the hospital, Doris and Sam returned home in silence. Doris prepped that night, taking the laxatives as prescribed and becoming increasingly disconcerted by the blood present in the toilet bowl with each laxative-induced bowel movement. She slept fitfully, wishing the morning would arrive quickly and she could get on with the colonoscopy. They arrived at the hospital outpatient center promptly at 6:30 the following morning. Doris was escorted to a changing room at 7 A.M., and by 7:30 she was in the procedure suite, IV in arm and fading into sleep. She recalled little else of the morning's events despite Sam's prompting her about their conversation with Dr. K. in the recovery room. Sam recapitulated the discussion: Dr. K. said he saw a growth about 6 inches into the rectum; the growth was bleeding; the growth's appearance was suspicious; he feared it was a cancerous tumor; he wasn't able to remove the growth but he was able to perform multiple biopsies and cauterize it to stop the bleeding; the pathologist should complete the review of the biopsy specimens in two days; even if the pathologist's analysis reveals a BENIGN growth, not MALIGNANT or cancerous, surgery would be needed to remove it since it had bled and it could not be removed in its entirety through the scope; he was recommending she see a colorectal surgeon.

Sam must have repeated the conversation a dozen times over the course of the day to concerned family and friends. Doris heard Sam repeat the details so many times she believed she was actually beginning to remember the conversation with Dr. K. in the recovery room.

They had been referred to Dr. Armstrong, whom friends affirmed was a topnotch colorectal surgeon. Doris and Sam met Dr. Armstrong several days later. He was direct and to the point, but his explanation was also delivered with warmth and compassion. In a nutshell the biopsies revealed a malignant tumor that he referred to as an ADENOCARCINOMA of the rectum. More testing was still needed to evaluate the full extent of the cancer problem. Surgery would be needed to remove the cancer but surgery by itself would likely not offer the best chance of cure. Receiving chemotherapy and radiation treatments before surgery would give Doris the best chance of cure. He recommended Doris see both a MEDICAL ONCOLOGIST and a RADIATION ONCOLOGIST. He called the specialists while Doris and Sam sat across from him in his office. They listened as he spouted off the medical jargon explaining Doris's case. The words became a jumble of encrypted code as they heard CT SCAN, STAGE II, T3, LAR, until they were too confused to continue listening.

Dr. Armstrong confirmed that Doris would see the radiation oncologist, Dr. Drake, a week later on Tuesday morning and the medical oncologist, Dr. Feinberg, Tuesday afternoon. This Thursday she would undergo a CT scan of the abdomen and pelvis, and on Friday she would return to his office to undergo an ULTRA-SOUND of the tumor. By week's end Doris will have seen five doctors, undergone more tests than she can remember, and experienced enough rectal exams to fill a lifetime. Doris and Sam left Dr. Armstrong's office dazed and confused, scared but still in remarkably good humor. Sam tried to lighten up the mood when he quipped, "I wonder how many doctors it takes to change a light bulb?"

I met Doris and Sam for the first time that Tuesday afternoon. I had spoken to all of her physicians except Dr. Drake whom I had planned to speak with after our visit.

I have been seeing couples like Doris and Sam every week for nearly 20 years. I share their anguish; I see their pain. They had suffered through a week of anxiety, fear, and emotional suffering that was to continue for possibly another week until the results of testing would dictate final treatment recommendations. Despite family and friends, the physician consultations, books, and the Internet, patients like Doris and Sam remain in the isolation of the unknown, their minds inextricably fixating on the worst-case scenario. Doris and Sam and the tens of thousands of people like them cannot find comfort or calm their irrational fear until they understand the physiologic and biologic processes related to this odyssey. They need time to digest the myriad of pieces of information thrown at them, and they need the fact filtered from the fiction. They need the information accessible to digest at their pace, not in the 30 minutes allotted to them in the doctor's office. This book provides that information. This book is for every Doris and Sam, their children and siblings, their caring friends, and their parents. It is for the more than 150,000 newly diagnosed colon cancer patients this year and the millions of men and women living with a diagnosis of colon cancer in the United States. It is also a book for those at risk of colon cancer, which includes all of us over 50 years of age, as colon cancer is a disease which can be prevented and if found early, cured.

Let me explain to you the way I explain to my patients, like Doris and Sam, what happened to her body that resulted in a colorectal cancer diagnosis. I begin, as does the cancer, with a single cell.

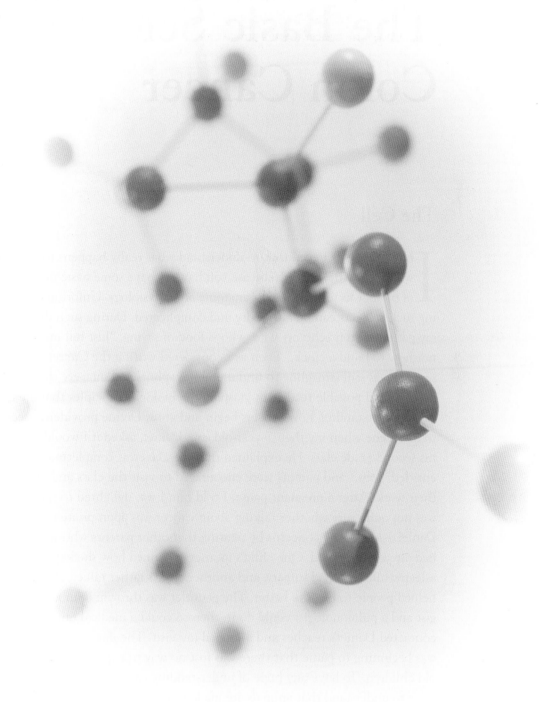

Chapter One

The Basic Science of Colon Cancer

The Cell

I have always believed that to understand what really happens to the body when it is stricken with disease you have to have some basic understanding of biology as well as human anatomy and physiology. Unfortunately, discussing such subjects can be rather dry and complicated. During such discussions my patients often echo my wife, who is fond of saying, "Just tell me the time, not how to build a clock." Even as I considered writing the *Cancer Answers* series, I was still struggling to find useful metaphors and imagery to assist my patients and possible readers in grasping the biologic principles that are critical to understanding how cancers begin and grow. Divine providence seemed to intervene when my then 7-year-old son, Daniel, asked if I would speak to his second-grade class. He explained that the class was completing a study unit entitled "Jobs," and parents were encouraged to visit the class and talk about their work. After a pregnant pause, I told him I was delighted to speak, but I was not quite sure whether talking about cancer was appropriate for 7 year olds. Daniel assuaged my concerns by relating that other parents who were physicians had already presented. One child's mother explained how she kept sick people asleep while they had surgery, and another child's father talked about how he helped people to breathe better. The gauntlet was thrown: if an anesthesiologist and a pulmonologist could do it, then so could a medical oncologist. I contacted Daniel's teacher and arranged my visit. The day approached, and I was beginning to panic that there was just no way to explain cancer to 7-year-old children. To have any hope of understanding cancer and its treatment, you have to understand that animals are made from cells, that cells can transform

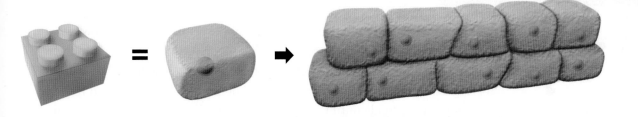

Figure 1-1 The Lego—the Perfect Metaphor for the Cell

and grow out of control, and that medicines are available that can kill these transformed, bad-behaving cells without harming the good cells that keep us alive. Unfortunately, these kids were in second grade and did not even know what a cell was.

I went to Daniel's bedroom to confess my dilemma. Daniel was on the floor with his Legos splayed about him. When I saw the hundreds of Legos in every color, shape, and size joined in various ways to create cars, houses, and planes, I had an epiphany. The Lego was the perfect metaphor for a cell (Figure 1-1).

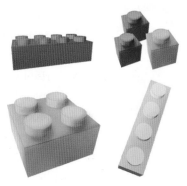

Figure 1-2: Assorted Legos

In Legoland, the Lego is the basic building block. Hundreds of different types of Legos when appropriately combined can create an infinite variety of structures. You can take Legos of just one variety and stack them side by side and up and down to create a wall. Add two windows and a door, and create the completed front wall of a house. After a child builds three sidewalls and secures them with a floor and a roof, the house takes on a recognizable appearance. Eureka, my problem was solved (Figure 1-2).

I explained to Daniel that while the Lego is the basic building block of Legoland, the cell is the basic building block of organic life (living creatures). The cell is called the origin of life because animals grow from a single cell made by the joining of sperm and egg. One cell gives rise to the billions of cells that make the complete animal. Like Legos, the billions of cells are not identical in appearance but rather fall into a few hundred different types: hair cells, skin cells, blood cells, etc. (Figure 1-3).

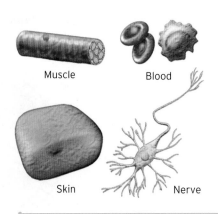

Muscle Blood

Skin Nerve

Figure 1-3: Assorted Cells

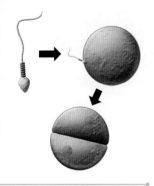

Figure 1-4:
The Origin of Life

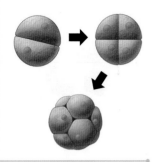

Figure 1-5:
Cellular Division

The formation of the human body, like any mammal's body, begins with the meeting of a sperm and an egg. The sperm fertilizes the egg, which creates the first cell, the beginning of a human body (Figure 1-4). This cell then divides to make two cells. Two cells divide to make four, and then those cells continue to divide until there is a cluster of cells (Figure 1-5). Initially, all of the cells in the cluster are identical. Next these identical cells begin a process in which they become the more than 200 different types of cells that make the human body complete. This process is called DIFFERENTIATION; the cells differentiate or become different types. This early developing human is called an EMBRYO.

The process of differentiation in the developing embryo begins with these clustered cells organizing into three layers: an outer layer called ECTODERM, an inner layer called ENDODERM, and a middle layer called MESODERM. These three layers of cells are in turn encased in a layer of cells that will give rise to the placenta. The outer of these three layers, ectoderm, differentiates into skin and nerve cells. The middle layer, mesoderm, differentiates into blood, muscle, and bone cells. The inner layer, endoderm, differentiates into the cells that comprise all of the body's organs (Figure 1-6).

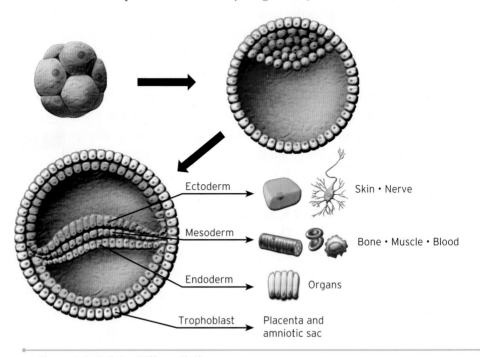

Ectoderm — Skin • Nerve

Mesoderm — Bone • Muscle • Blood

Endoderm — Organs

Trophoblast — Placenta and amniotic sac

Figure 1-6: Cellular Differentiation

Imagine Legoland being alive. In the beginning, there was one small, rectangular, white Lego. Then there were a bunch of small, rectangular, white Legos; then white Legos morphed into three groups—white, red, and blue rectangles.

Primitively speaking, all of your body's organ cells begin with the endoderm layer: they have a common origin and are structurally similar. This is a very important point, as we will later see. As these primitive cells further differentiate and mature, their structure and function assume that of adult cells. Mature cells progress from individual cells to sheets of cells. The sheets of cells then organize to form TISSUES. Different types of tissues combine to form organs. Finally, the organs are arranged within a musculoskeletal framework supported by a circulatory and nervous system.

Returning to our Legoland metaphor, the white, blue, and red Legos have now morphed into hundreds of different types. There are billions of each type, trillions of Legos in all. Some Legos have been assembled into a wall (like sheets of cells forming tissues). Doors and windows have been added to the wall to make the front of a house (like an organ), and roofs, floors, walls, and more have been organized to make a complete house (like a complete human being).

Daniel was an attentive and courteous listener as I expounded gleefully, progressing from Legos and cells to cancer and treatment. When I finished my diatribe, gratified to have found the long-sought metaphor, I asked Daniel what he thought. He said that he liked the Lego part but that I definitely needed to bring some kind of neat machine, like the breathing thing with the balls that go up and down that the lung doctor demonstrated. Also, I needed to bring a giveaway such as gloves or masks or maybe pencils with my name on it. I left Daniel's room defeated, feeling small and humbled. I went to my office with hopes of finding something appropriate to give 15 second graders, mired in thought of what kind of cancer machine I could demonstrate.

The Colon: Normal Structure And Function

Doris and Sam were among the first patients to see my Legos demonstration, and it was a success. Not only did they not think I was crazy, but it helped them to understand cells. The next step was to explain why humans have colons and what kinds of cells comprise them.

Unlike the Legos that I have been using for illustration, cells not only have structure, they also have function and are alive. To stay alive, cells must eat and breathe; blood provides the oxygen and nourishment. The body, like the cells that comprise it, also needs to eat and breathe. The food that's ingested for nourishment has to be broken down or DIGESTED into essential nutrients (fats, carbohydrates, and proteins) so they can be absorbed into the blood and transported to the cells in need. The organ system that facilitates the digestion and absorption of nutrients is referred to as the GASTROINTESTINAL SYSTEM or GI TRACT (Figure 1-7).

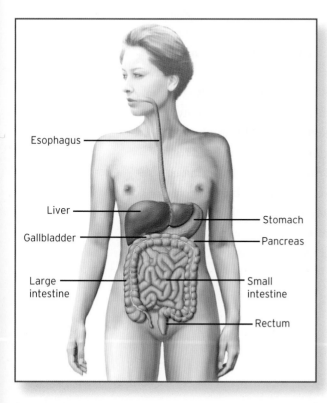

Figure 1-7: Gastrointestinal System

Esophagus

Liver

Gallbladder

Large intestine

Stomach

Pancreas

Small intestine

Rectum

The colon and rectum are key components of the GI tract (with the small INTESTINES they comprise the colloquially referred to BOWEL that gives rise to BOWEL MOVEMENTS). The basic biology and function of the colon and rectum may be better understood if we understand what happens to the food we eat as it passes through the digestive organs. The food entering the mouth is met with saliva, a mildly acidic liquid that also contains chemicals called DIGESTIVE ENZYMES. The saliva production was triggered in the brain by the thought, sight, and smell of food. The digestive enzymes and acid in the saliva, in conjunction with chewing, begin the digestive process. When chewed food is swallowed it is transported to the STOMACH through the muscular tube called the ESOPHAGUS. The muscular component is present throughout the organs of the GI tract as the nutrient-rich food and later nutrient-poor waste is propelled forward by a sequential squeezing motion, a process called PERISTALSIS (imagine a mouse traveling through a snake). Once in the stomach, the minimally digested food is exposed to a harsh environment with greater acidity and more digestive enzymes. The food will reside for a time in this acidic and enzyme-rich milieu to continue the process of decomposition. The food is prevented from re-entering the esophagus by a muscular valve called the ESOPHAGEAL SPHINCTER, and it is held in the stomach by another muscular valve called the PYLORIC SPHINCTER, which controls its exit.

Immediately upon exiting the stomach, the partially digested food enters the SMALL INTESTINE. In the first of three portions of the small intestine, the nutrient-enzyme-acid mix is augmented by more digestive enzymes from the PANCREAS as well as BILE from the LIVER. The bile is stored in the GALLBLAD-DER, unless gallbladder disease, usually stones, has previously necessitated surgical removal. In the presence of the many enzymes, bile, and denaturing acid, the nutrient-rich slurry is reduced to its most basic components of proteins, carbohydrates, and fats. In the 30 or so feet of intestine (divided into three anatomically distinct sections: DUODENUM, JEJUNUM, and ILEUM) the body uses MUCOSA (specialized cells lining the inside surface) to ABSORB or take in the nutrients from the digested food. The loops and loops of small intestine end in the lower right quadrant of the abdomen where the small intestine or UPPER GI TRACT transitions into the COLON, also referred to as the LOWER GI TRACT, LARGE BOWEL, and LARGE INTESTINE. Two distinct anatomic structures, the APPENDIX and the CECUM, identify this transition region at the end of the ileum and the start of the colon. The nutrient-rich food consumed hours ago has now traversed the esophagus, stomach, and 30 feet of small intestine. During this journey, food was depleted of nutrients leaving only water and waste, like indigestible plant fiber, to be propelled through the colon via peristalsis.

Similar to the small intestine, the colon is divided into sections or segments. There are five segments in all. The first segment, or ASCENDING COLON, acquired its name because when one is standing, the material within it, waste and water, is propelled up or ascends from the lower right to the upper right abdominal quadrant. To use the correct anatomical-speak, the ascending colon transports waste and water from the ileum to the TRANSVERSE COLON, the second portion of the colon. The transition from ascending to transverse colon is marked by a 90-degree turn just below the liver, an anatomic refer-

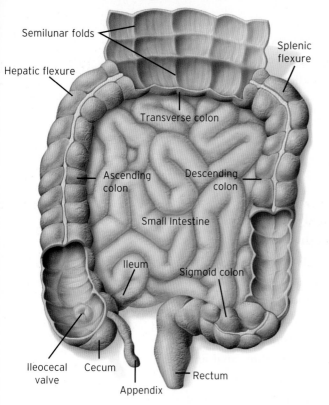

Figure 1-8: The Colon and Rectum

ence point referred to as the HEPATIC FLEXURE. The transverse segment of the colon crosses the upper abdomen from right to left. In the upper left abdominal quadrant, the colon once again takes a 90-degree turn anatomically referred to as the SPLENIC FLEXURE, which marks the next transition. The colon then descends (if one is standing) in a straight line toward the left hip; hence this third portion of the colon is called the DESCENDING COLON. The end of the descending colon, just above the left hip, is the fourth transition point. Here the colon leaves the abdominal cavity and enters the PELVIC CAVITY, taking on an s-shape to curve around other anatomic structures (like the bladder). The name of this s-shaped segment comes from the Greek letter, sigma, and is thus called the SIGMOID COLON (Figure 1-8).

Throughout this journey, which follows the periphery of the abdominal cavity, the specialized mucosal cells lining the interior of the colon have been busy removing the one critical nutrient not claimed by the small intestine, water. By the time the digested food reaches the cecum, all of the nutrients have been resorbed, leaving only waste and water. After the entire colon has been traversed and the water reclaimed, all that remains is waste. As the sigmoid colon enters the PELVIS, it transitions once again, this time into the RECTUM, a reservoir for waste. Another muscular valve or sphincter permits voluntary evacuation of waste from the rectal vault, a process technically referred to as DEFECATION. This valve is called the ANAL SPHINCTER. An intact anal sphincter permits voluntary defecation referred to as BOWEL CONTINENCE, but if the sphincter is damaged then waste leaks uncontrollably, referred to as BOWEL or FECAL INCONTINENCE. The anal sphincter is the anatomic landmark for the final transition connecting the rectum to the outside, through an orifice or opening called the ANUS.

At this point in my presentation, I could tell Doris and Sam were perplexed by my insistence that we take this virtual tour of the GI tract. I explained that to understand the location of the cancer, its cause, the therapy needed for cure, and possible side effects of treatment, it was necessary to understand the anatomy. They refocused as I posed a question. "When you look at yourself in the mirror you might distinguish your chest from your abdomen but can you distinguish your abdomen from your pelvis?" I offered, "You might get a bit of help figuring out where your pelvis is positioned by sitting down: The part of the body that you saw in the mirror when you were standing but is now obstructed from view by your legs is your pelvis." The PELVIC or PERINEAL CAVITY is anatomically distinct from the ABDOMINAL or PERITONEAL CAVITY. The abdominal cavity contains most of the colon, all the small intestines, and the other organs of digestion as well as the liver, spleen, and kidneys. The pelvic cavity is a basin or bowl-shaped cavity created by your hipbones and lower backbone that forms the end of your body's trunk. The organs encased and protected by this bony cavity include the rectum, the bladder, the male prostate, and the female uterus, ovaries, and fallopian tubes. The skin surface between the thighs, where the rectum via the anus, the bladder via the urethra, and the genitals communicate with the outside is referred to as the PERINEUM.

Having reviewed the entire gastrointestinal tract from appetite to anus and learning the differences between the abdomen and pelvis Doris and Sam were ready to understand the relationships of the colon and rectum to the rest of the three-dimensional abdomino-pelvic anatomy. To understand these relationships, visualization techniques will help but, first we need some directional keys. Doctors realized early on that since the body is three dimensional, describing up or down can get confusing, i.e., when standing, up might be toward the head and down might be toward the toe, but when lying down, up may be toward the belly button and down may be toward the buttocks. Rather than up/down or front/back, the anatomy teachers came up with a more accurate map key for the body. Toward the head is referred to as CEPHALAD. Toward the feet is referred to as CAUDAD. Toward the front of the body (belly button, chin) is ANTERIOR while toward the back (spine, buttocks) is POSTERIOR. When we describe something located toward the midline we refer to it as MEDIAL, and that which is located away from the midline is referred to as LATERAL. Finally we need a way to explain positions relative to a point of anatomic interest. Regarding a segment of colon, the end that is closer to the small intestine is PROXIMAL, whereas the end that is closer to the anus is DISTAL; e.g., the rectum is distal to the sigmoid colon but proximal to the anus (Figure 1-9).

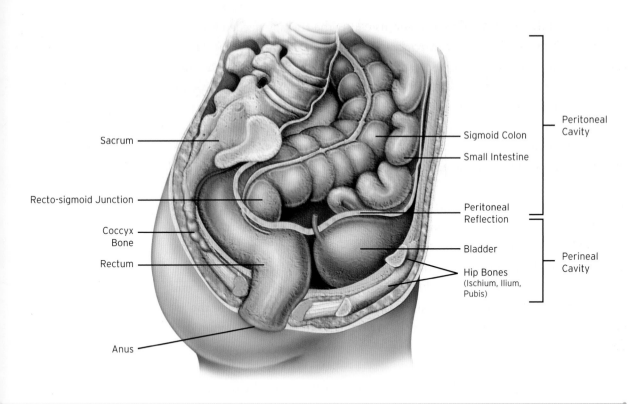

Figure 1-9: Abdominal and Pelvic Cavities

Our next task is to try to visualize the abdomen from top to bottom or cephalad to caudad. You might think of the colon as a 6-foot length of garden hose lying under the skin and muscle of your belly or, in correct anatomic speak, the anterior abdominal wall. It's positioned in a horseshoe shaped arch with the points down or caudad. The horseshoe outlines the periphery of the abdomen with the right arm of the horseshoe (ascending colon) beginning just above the right hip bone, the arch of the horseshoe (transverse colon) following along the diaphragm and the left arm of the horseshoe (descending colon) parallel to the right ending at the left hip bone. Lying within the borders created by the horseshoe is a layer of connective tissue like the webbed pocket of a baseball glove, called the MESENTERY (Figure 1-10).

Let's now try to image the abdomen front to back, or in correct anatomic speak, anterior to posterior. The colon and intestines sit against the anterior abdominal wall in the anterior abdominal compartment. Behind or posterior to the colon and intestines lie the kidneys and ureters. Posterior to the kidneys lay the major blood vessels of the trunk, the main artery AORTA and the main vein VENA CAVA. The posterior wall of the abdomen is defined by the backbone and supporting muscles.

The sigmoid colon arises from the left end of the horseshoe coursing both caudad, toward the crotch (not an accepted anatomic term), as well as posterior, toward the backbone, as it leaves the abdomen and enters the pelvis. The rectum resides strictly within the pelvis. This completes our lesson in gross anatomy. It's gross not because it's icky but because we're referring to the anatomy as it looks to the unaided eye before it's dissected and placed under a microscope (just like your paycheck is gross before it's dissected with taxes and deductions).

With the images of the gross anatomy of the gastrointestinal tract now etched in your memory we are ready to look beneath the surface at the structures not visible to the naked eye. We begin our discussion of microscopic anatomy by visualizing the tissues that comprise the colon and rectum.

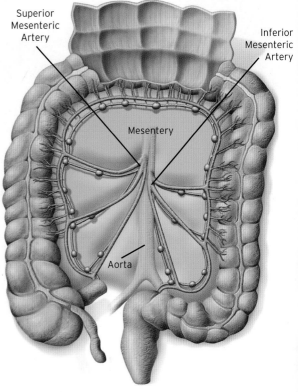

Figure 1-10: Colon and Rectum with Mesentery and Circulation

All of our organs have specialized cells that perform the unique functions that define them. There are specialized cells in the breast that make milk, there are specialized cells in the pancreas that produce insulin and digestive enzymes, and there are specialized cells in the intestines that permit the absorption of nutrients. These specialized cells comprise the GLANDULAR TISSUE of the organ and require a host of other supporting tissues necessary for their function. The specialized cells of the colon permit its unique operation to reclaim water.

Under low-power magnification, the microscope reveals the colon not to be a simple 5- to 6-foot garden-hose-like tube but rather a complex multilayered cylindrical structure. Three main layers are apparent, the outer protective membrane or SEROSA, the more substantial muscular layer or MUSCULARIS that facilitates peristalsis, and the innermost layer or MUCOSA, which is comprised

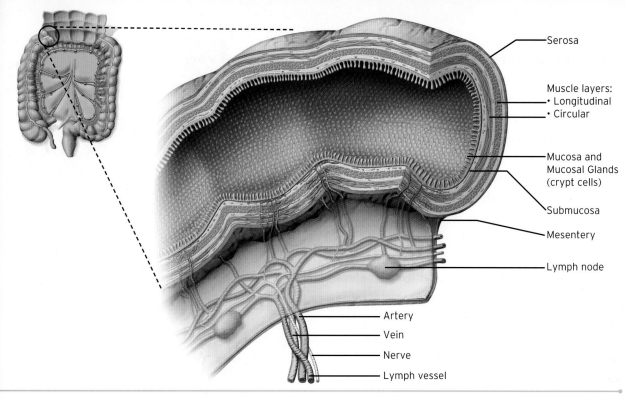

Figure 1-11: Low Power Magnification of the Colon

of the specialized glandular tissue that facilitates the absorption of water. The muscle layer creates an appearance of centipede-like segmentation called HAUS-TRA, visible both on the outside and inside of the colon, but the colon remains hollow throughout (Figure 1-11).

The diseases referred to as colon cancer develop in the mucosal layer of the colon. Both men and women have colons and are equally exposed to the agents that promote colonic mucosal cell transformation to cancer. Before we can begin to understand how and why the mucosal cells transform we need to delve a bit deeper into the microscopic anatomy of the colon. We must visualize the cellular layers that permit the colon its unique function of water reclamation.

The mucosal lining appears smooth to the unaided eye but under the microscope we see that the mucosa is more like a brush with tightly packed, short bristles. The spaces or valleys between the bristles of the brush are called CRYPTS where the water reclamation work occurs. The waste and water are propelled by peristalsis across the top of the bristles of the brush allowing the water to collect in the crypts where it can be absorbed by the CRYPT CELLS. Below the layer of crypt cells lie the small blood vessels into which the absorbed water is transferred.

Doris and Sam were patient listeners as I conducted this lesson in anatomy with my words and pencil drawings. They were ready for the next lesson when I would explain how these normal colon crypt cells are transformed into cancer.

Carcinogenesis

Throughout your lifetime cells are continuously injured and repaired. Bruises, scrapes, cuts, burns, infections, chapped lips, and tongues burned by pizza cheese and hot coffee are a sample of the myriad of everyday cellular injuries that you experience. Your body has the remarkable ability to repair this cellular damage and does so in a constant, ongoing process. Some cellular damage is below the surface, caused by the tobacco smoke that we inhale, the chemicals in the food that we eat, the radiation from the sun, and the internal (natural), physical, chemical, and hormonal stresses that are part and parcel of being alive. Sometimes, if the injuries are chronic or recurrent, or if there is a genetic predisposing defect, the body is unable to repair the cellular injury. The body's failure or inability to repair cellular injury can lead to cancer. The process by which the failed repair of cellular injury leads to cancer is called CARCINOGENESIS.

In the beginning of this chapter, I mentioned that all of the body's specialized organ tissue has a common origin in the cells of the endoderm of the developing embryo. As these primitive cells mature, they retain certain common features, giving organ tissue a similar appearance under the microscope. The microscopic appearance is often referred to as GLANDULAR, which means something different than what you might think. To a PATHOLOGIST, glandular tissue refers to a group of cells that are organized so that they can either take in nutrients (absorb) or release chemicals needed to maintain normal body function (secrete). The cell type common to these glandular tissues is called an EPITHELIAL CELL. The epithelial cells are flat where they connect the organs to the outside, such as at the mouth and anus; are cube-shaped in the organs that are secretory, such as the breast, prostate, and pancreas; and are an elongated cube or column shaped in the organs that absorb nutrients, such as the colon

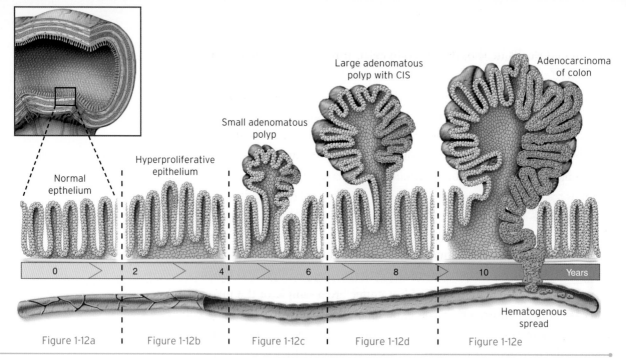

Figure 1-12a–e: High Power Magnification of Colonic Mucosa with Time Sequence of Carcinogenesis

and small intestine. When flat epithelial cells transform into cancer, they are called SQUAMOUS CELL CARCINOMA. When cuboidal or columnar epithelial cells transform into cancer, they are called ADENOCARCINOMA.

The glandular tissue of the colon is comprised of the colonic mucosa and its crypt cells (Figure 1-12a). Researchers have begun to unravel the mystery of the genetic, molecular, and cellular changes that lead to the carcinogenesis of colonic mucosal tissue. As I explain later in Chapter 1, these injuries are not superficial and are not on the surface of the cell. Rather, these changes occur deep within the guts of the cell, in its nucleus and its DNA, changing the cell's appearance, behavior, and very essence. They can turn a cell from a well-behaved and orderly Dr. Jekyll into Mr. Hyde, wreaking havoc and chaos. The process of transformation from Jekyll to Hyde is predictable, often slow, but relentless.

The transformation of colonic mucosal cells into cancer, is referred to as ADENOCARCINOMA OF THE COLON. The process begins with the physical and chemical stress on the mucosal cells, as they function continuously to reclaim water from the food we ingest. These chemical stresses may come from CAR-CINOGENS in the food we eat, from the bile acids that assist in the digestion of food, and/or from the bacteria that live within us. These stresses lead to irritation and then injury of the mucosal cells. If the body is unable to repair the injured cells, new cells are added to the injured ones, resulting in an overgrowth of mucosal cells, which is called HYPERPROLIFERATIVE (Figure 1-12b).

As the mucosal cells continue to overgrow, they become unstable, altering their appearance and behavior. The cells become larger and less uniform, their growth pattern less organized. Continued stress, cellular injury, and repair process mistakes result in what are called MUTATIONS (physical changes in cellular DNA described in more detail later in this chapter), which lead to the creation of more aggressive cells. These more aggressive cells may so overgrow that they create a mound. The mound may be flat or it may be mushroom-like. The cellular mound, called a POLYP, may become large enough that it can be felt on examination (if in the rectum), interfere with passing feces, bleed, or be visualized through an endo-scope. At this point, pathologists call the overgrowth ADENOMATOUS (Figure 1-12c). Additional mutations may result in these adenomatous polyps developing CIS (CARCINOMA IN-SITU) the earliest form of cancer (Figure 1-12d).

Unfortunately, patients do not always experience or observe changes in their stool caliber or color, observe blood in the stool, develop symptomatic anemia from bleeding, or undergo routine screening exams (discussed in detail in Chapter 2). If CIS remains undetected, the next cellular event that can occur is an even more aggressive change. These unstable, mutated mucosal crypt cells that have met the first criterion of cancer by their pattern of overgrowth no longer respect the boundary of the mucosal layer. They invade or infiltrate through the mucosa (visualize a tree root growing through the street or sidewalk). This IN-FILTRATING tumor, or INVASIVE colonic adenocarcinoma, is the most advanced form of cancer within the colon and or rectum (Figure 1-12e).

The more I explained to Doris and Sam, the more questions they had. Doris was confused: She didn't smoke, she ate a well-balanced diet and she exercised everyday. Sam chimed in, "She eats like a bird, how could she have developed a cancer in her rectum?" I advised a deep breath and patience because I was just about to explain how normal, everyday stress could cause cellular injury and initiate the cascade of events that result in cancer. In order to understand the how and why of carcinogenesis, one needs to understand the inner workings of a cell—its GENETIC CODE.

Genetics

All human cells have a similar design: an outer membrane covering a gelatinous liquid cytoplasm within which is a central core structure, the nucleus. The image is that of a Tootsie Roll Pop where the wrapper is the cell membrane, the lollypop candy is the cytoplasm, and the Tootsie Roll is the nucleus (Figure 1-13). Within the nucleus resides the blueprint or operating code of not only the cell but also of the entire organism.

Like computer software written in special binary code, the operating code of living organisms is written in a special language called DNA, which is actually a chemical code comprised of four characters called NUCLEOSIDE BASES. DNA is a unique code language that, once translated, instructs the cell to build PROTEINS. Proteins are the cell's machines that bring food into the cell, remove waste from the cell, repair the cell after injury, prepare the cell for growth and division, etc.

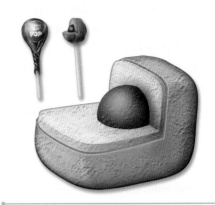

Figure 1-13: The Cell as a Tootsie Pop

Like many other types of machines that we are more familiar with, proteins may have many different functions but are all structurally related. Automobiles, tractors, speedboats, and helicopters are very different forms of transportation but are all propelled by an internal combustion engine. Refrigerators, blenders, washers, and coffee grinders are very different appliances, but they are all powered by an electric motor. Computers, cell phones, digital cameras, and CD players perform different functions, but they are all controlled by a microprocessor chip. Like each of these examples of inorganic machines, proteins are the workhorses of organic machines and the cells that comprise them. The blueprint for each protein is encrypted in the DNA code.

By definition, a code must be broken or translated for the encrypted message to be understood. The DNA message for protein building requires not only translation, but it must also get transported from the nucleus to the cytoplasm where the proteins are manufactured. The translation and subsequent transport of the encrypted DNA message is facilitated by another nucleoside base language called RNA. The DNA message is translated to RNA, which leaves the nucleus and travels to the cytoplasm where it docks with a structure called a RIBOSOME, the protein-manufacturing factory.

The chemical building blocks of proteins are called AMINO ACIDS. The amino acids are chemically linked one to another according to the instructions of the DNA message. Let me try to summarize in a single statement: *Amino acids in the cytoplasm are assembled into proteins by the ribosome under the direction of an RNA message, which is the translation of a DNA code sequence from within the nucleus* (Figure 1-14).

A complete DNA sequence that encodes a protein is called a GENE. Genes are clustered into long strands of DNA called CHROMOSOMES, which are made even longer because these genes are also separated from one another by non-message base sequences. There are 46 chromosomes in a normal human cell, 23 contributed by the father via the sperm and 23 contributed by the mother via the egg. The chromosomes are arranged in 23 pairs. Scientists now believe that there are between 20,000 and 40,000 genes necessary for human life, making it likely that there are approximately 1,000 to 2,000 genes per chromosome pair.

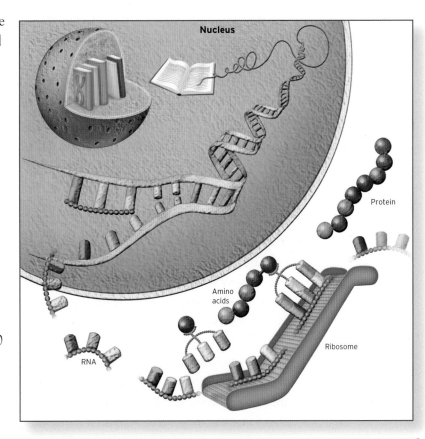

Figure 1-14: The Biochemical Basis of Life: DNA-RNA-Protein. Amino acids in the cytoplasm are assembled into proteins by the ribosome under the direction of an RNA message, which is the translation of a DNA code sequence from within the nucleus. Every cell in the body has the complete manual of information (genome) stored in its library (nucleus).

Think of this genetic operating system or GENOME as the body's complete information encyclopedia or better still, the body's owner's manual. Everything needed to build, operate, and repair the body is written in the manual, a copy residing in each cell. The encyclopedic size owner's manual is comprised of 23 volumes (chromosome pairs), each 1,000–2,000 chapters long (genes) composed in a four-character code language (DNA) requiring billions of characters (nucleoside bases) in all. *Every cell in the body has the complete manual of information (genome) stored in its library (nucleus)*, but only certain volumes are off the shelf at any one time, opened to specific chapters as the genetic needs dictate. Genes for hair color would not be turned on in blood cells, and genes to produce HEMOGLOBIN would not be turned on in hair cells. Beginning in the embryo and throughout cellular differentiation, fetal maturation, growth, and development, messages are turned on and off in a complex system of signals and responses. For the messages and signaling to work properly, every cell needs to have its billions of characters (nucleoside bases) in the correct sequence, ready for the moment when one of the volumes is taken off the shelf and opened to a chapter to be translated. A mistake in a base sequence is called a MUTATION.

Mutations can occur in a variety of ways. Let's use that encyclopedic owner's manual metaphor to illustrate the point. Sometimes information passed on from a parent is incorrect, causing some of the chapters to have wrong information. Such genetic mutations are called HEREDITARY MUTATIONS. Sometimes there is a misprint at the factory (embryo or fetus), leading to incorrect information in some of the chapters. Such genetic mutations are called CONGENITAL MUTATIONS. Most commonly, the original information and printing are correct, but from years of use and handling, print becomes smudged, paper stained, or pages torn, leading to incorrect messages. Such genetic mutations are called ACQUIRED MUTATIONS.

Genetic defects or mutations that cause a cell to reproduce uncontrollably and invade surrounding structures are what cause cancer. Many forms of cellular injury like those caused by chemicals and radiation lead to the types of mutations that cause carcinogenesis. Acquired mutations rarely occur from a single insult but rather from repeated insult and injury like years of tobacco use, chronic irritation from fecal waste, decades of cyclic hormonal stress, or just living. Thus, all cancers are consequences of genetic mutations, but few, approximately 10%, are hereditary. Most cancers are the result of acquired genetic mutations (Figure 1-15).

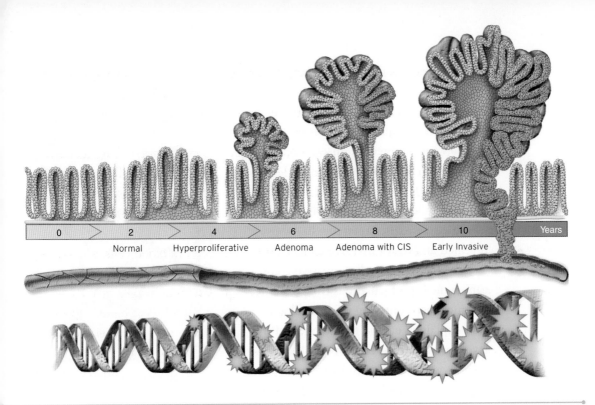

0	2	4	6	8	10	Years
Normal	Hyperproliferative	Adenoma	Adenoma with CIS	Early Invasive		

Figure 1-15 Polyp Evolution as a Series of Mutation Events

Was Doris's cancer hereditary? Neither Doris's mother, father, brother, nor sister had a history of colon or rectum cancer. She had a single benign colon polyp seen and removed at her first colonoscopy but that was more than 10 years ago. Since then, two colonoscopies had been clear. She also now understood that her age at diagnosis, more than 70 years, suggested that her risk of having a hereditary colorectal cancer was very low, a relief as she now thought about her children. So if her cancer wasn't hereditary then what caused it?

Colon cancer, like the majority of adult cancers, most often occurs in the sixth, seventh, and eighth decades of life and is predominantly the result of acquired mutations brought about by years of cellular stress and injury. The transformation to cancer is slow, taking years or decades as gene after gene is mutated until one day the mutations are extensive enough to meet the criteria that define cancer. The most serious mutations are those that confer on a cell the behaviors of invading surrounding structures and spreading through the BLOOD and LYMPH circulations. This was my next topic to discuss with Doris and Sam.

Invasion and Metastases

Doris's normal colon exam just a little more than four years ago, the recent onset of rectal bleeding, and the fact that she felt perfectly well caused her to be optimistic that her cancer was found early, before it was invasive. Unfortunately, the biopsy revealed an area of invasive cancer cells (Figure 1-16). What makes invasive colon cancer more problematic is the possibility of cancer cells entering into the blood. As I explained earlier, the colon, and the layers of tissue that comprise it, is a living organ composed of cells. Every cell must have a blood supply to survive. Therefore, supporting the mucosal tissue are blood vessels sending off small branches that not only nourish each of the living cells that make up the mucosal layer but also retrieve the water reclaimed by the crypt cells. As the invasive cancer grows through or infiltrates the layers beneath the mucosa, root-like projections of tumor may also grow through or infiltrate the wall of nearby blood vessels. Once exposed to the bloodstream, cancer cells may break free from the growing cluster (tumor) gaining access to the blood circulation as it flows through the colon (Figure 1-17).

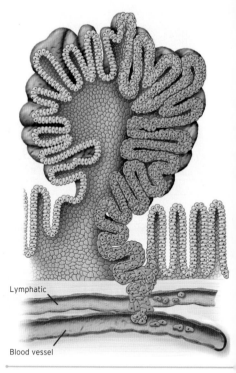

Figure 1-16: Vascular and Lymphatic Invasion

If individual cancer cells or cell clusters survive in the blood circulation, they may adhere to or anchor to the wall of a blood vessel anywhere in the body and there begin a new nest of growing cancer cells. This nest may then invade through the blood vessel wall (just as it originally invaded through the mucosa). The nest may then extend into the organ in which that blood vessel is located (the lung, the liver, etc.), forming a cancerous tumor in that organ (Figure 1-18). The nest of colon cancer cells anchored into a blood vessel of another organ where it then forms a cancerous tumor is what doctors call a METASTASIS (a similar process can occur within the lymph circulation of the colon, as explained in Chapter 3).

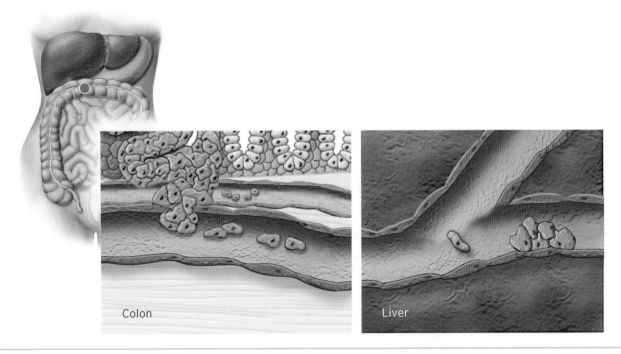

Figure 1-17: Downstream Adherence and Nesting of CirculatingTumor Cells

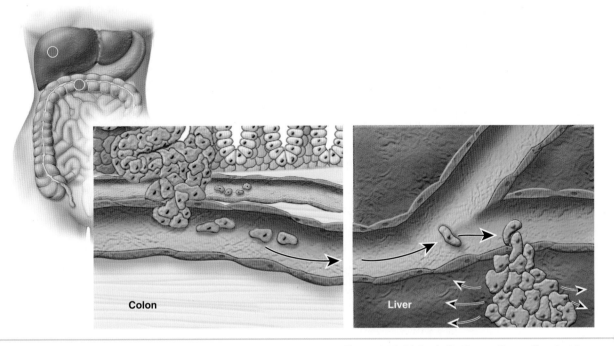

Figure 1-18: Metastatic Tumor Formation in Liver

The overriding concern for the patients with infiltrating or invasive colon cancer, and the doctors who treat them, is whether colon cancer cells have escaped into the circulation and might develop into metastases. The mission of the medical oncologist, like me, is to determine the risk of metastases in order to either do something preemptively to destroy the escaping cells before they anchor, nest, and/or invade another organ (ADJUVANT THERAPY) or to treat the metastases if they can be identified or are readily apparent (METASTATIC THERAPY).

Fortunately for Doris, like most men and women who undergo regular colon cancer screening, if a cancer is diagnosed, even when that cancer is invasive, it is found in its early stages when cure is likely. *Three facts about colon cancer are worth enumerating here. Fact one, 90% of all colon cancers found during routine screening colonoscopies are cured. Fact two, 90% of colon cancers arise from acquired genetic mutations and occur in people over the age of 50, the age at which routine screening-colonoscopies should commence. Fact three, more than 80% of all colon cancers could be prevented or cured if all at risk individuals, which means everyone upon turning 50, underwent screening. The simple math is overwhelming. If routine colon cancer screening guidelines were followed, more than 80% of colon cancer deaths would be avoided.*

Unfortunately, some colon cancers, about 10%, arise in men and women under age 50 who have no known risk of hereditary colon cancer. Eric was such a patient. Let's move on to the next chapter as I introduce Eric. We will discuss the second most common presenting SYMPTOM of colon cancer, IRON DEFICIENCY ANEMIA, and the bleeding colonic tumors that are responsible. We'll catch up with Doris and Sam a bit later.

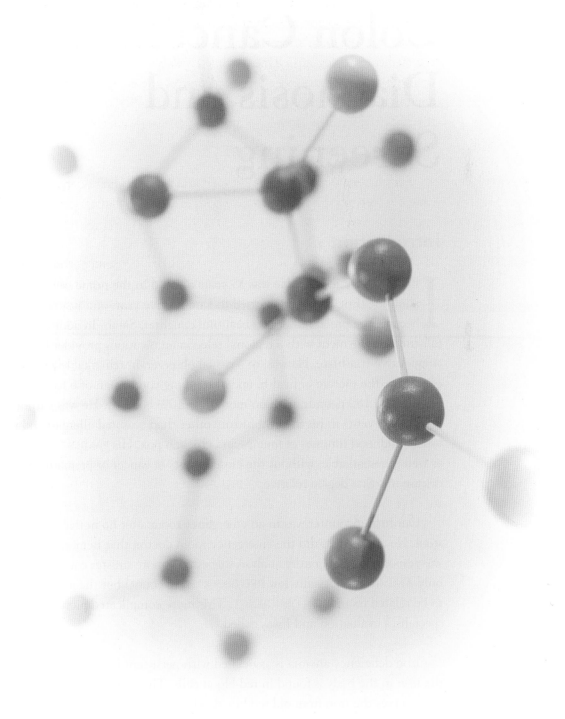

Chapter Two

Colon Cancer: Diagnosis and Screening

Introduction

I first met Eric in June. He was 35 years old and in the prime of his young adult life. Eric had been married to Kim for five years and just recently became the proud father of a beautiful daughter, Sarah. In addition to his full-time employment with a regional telecommunications provider he was a competitive triathlete. He was, to a casual observer, in remarkable physical condition, the picture of health, and a strapping young man of 6 feet, 2 inches. He weighed 180 pounds, with no more than 10% body fat. He was without any reportable events in his medical history other than seasonal allergies and the usual childhood illnesses of mumps and chicken pox. His FAMILY HISTORY was as well unremarkable, without the closet ghosts of cancer or premature heart disease in a first degree relative.

Our first encounter was in an emergency room after he noticed a bloody stool. He assumed, as did the emergency room doctor, that hemorrhoid bleeding was responsible. Laboratory analysis suggested a more sinister cause as he was not only ANEMIC (abnormally low RED BLOOD CELL count) but the anemia appeared to be related to an IRON DEFICIENCY. This more complicated picture warranted a specialist's evaluation and I was called.

Iron deficiency anemia is associated with persistent blood loss. Most of the iron in the body is found in red blood cells. The body is very efficient; it conserves the iron from old red blood cells and reutilizes it to build new red blood cells. Iron is also readily available from many types of food. In short, outside the nutritional demands of pregnancy, malnutrition, and rare malabsorption conditions, one doesn't become deficient in iron unless iron is lost; you only lose iron when you lose blood and it takes a lot of blood loss to result in iron deficiency.

When a large amount of blood is lost suddenly, referred to as an ACUTE BLEED, the blood loss is usually observed and it also produces symptoms, like lightheadedness and shortness of breath. However, when blood loss is slow and continuous, referred to as a CHRONIC BLEED, the bleeding is more insidious as the body compensates for the blood loss. A person may remain asymptomatic while becoming both iron deficient and anemic. Red blood cells survive, on average, only four months, necessitating continuous repletion. Without the necessary iron to build new red blood cells, the body's red blood cell count declines and the cells that are made do not achieve full size, resulting in the classically described MICROCYTIC (Latin for small cell) ANEMIA of iron deficiency. Iron deficiency anemia is quite common in young women as chronic, monthly menstrual blood loss causes loss of iron resulting in iron depletion. However, iron deficiency in an older, post-menopausal woman or in a man suggests a disease process.

Obviously, Eric didn't have menstrual blood loss. He had no history of gastrointestinal disease or surgery to suggest malabsorption. He was thin but not malnourished. He ate a normal diet with lots of iron-containing foods like red meat and green leafy vegetables. The only possible explanation for Eric's iron deficiency was that he had more bleeding than was evident in the ER doctor's notes. Eric swore that this was the first time he saw blood. Eric had no reason to lie. The only plausible explanation for his iron deficiency anemia was he was bleeding without knowing it. Hemorrhoid bleeding is always obvious as the blood from the rectum and anus will be seen in the toilet bowel and on the toilet paper. The only suitable explanation for Eric's unobserved or OCCULT BLOOD LOSS was chronic bleeding deep within the gastrointestinal tract. Before leaving the body, the blood was decomposing and mixing with fecal waste, masking its appearance.

Occult or hidden gastrointestinal blood loss is actually a common occurrence. In young men like Eric, iron deficiency anemia is most often associated with bleeding that results from irritation and/or ulceration of the stomach lining referred to as gastritis, gastric ulcer, or peptic ulcer. Even if Eric were bleeding from an asymptomatic case of gastritis or gastric ulcer this diagnosis wouldn't explain the bright red blood Eric saw in the toilet bowl. Blood from the stomach would have had to travel through 30 feet of small intestine and 6 feet of colon before getting to the toilet bowl and it certainly would have decomposed by then, appearing black and tarry not red. The bright red blood Eric observed meant that either there were two distinct problems associated with the bleeding (like a gastric ulcer and a hemorrhoid) or something more sinister was going on. That something would have to be a bleeding source that could cause both chronic asymptomatic occult blood loss as well as acute bright red blood loss. A bleeding source closer to the anus, in the colon, could have bled slowly and insidiously for a long time before the current episode of sudden severe bleeding that brought Eric to the emergency room. A colonoscopic evaluation by a GASTROENTEROLOGIST would be needed to sort this out.

The Polyp

Eric, like Doris, came to a physician's attention because he had observed a bloody bowel movement. Unfortunately, many patients with colon cancer never observe blood in the toilet bowl or a change in their stool. In this chapter we will review the clinical, laboratory, and DIAGNOSTIC IMAGING findings associated with colon cancer. We will also discuss the screening tests that can detect changes in the mucosal lining prior to the development of invasive cancer. Most importantly, we will take an in-depth look at the dreaded colonoscopy, the much maligned and irrationally feared but highly effective way to diagnose and more importantly prevent colon cancer. To understand the symptoms of anemia and change in bowel movements that may accompany a colon cancer; the value of screening tests, both laboratory and x-ray, that can detect precancerous changes; as well as procedures like sigmoidoscopy and colonoscopy, which can visualize abnormal colonic mucosa, we need to understand the POLYP.

To fully understand the polyp we need to visualize the mucosa of the colon as it overproduces cells in reaction to years of irritation from carcinogens, bacteria, and bile acids within the fecal waste. Like a sore that doesn't heal, cells become heaped upon cells as a cellular mound begins to emerge on the surface of the mucosal lining. As the mound grows it will become a visible protrusion (bump, mound, growth) arising from the mucosal surface that we call a polyp. Polyps are classified pathologically as (1) benign non-neoplastic overgrowths which include JUVENILE POLYPS and hyperplastic mucosal proliferations HYPERPLASTIC POLYPS, or (2) neoplastic overgrowths called ADENOMATOUS POLYPS. Only adenomatous polyps are clearly precancerous and only a minority, less than 1% will ever develop into cancer. Unfortunately, studies reveal that upwards of a third of middle-aged and elderly people have adenomatous polyps so the 1% rate of transformation results in more than 150,000 new colon cancers a year in the U.S. Polyps rarely produce any symptoms, remaining clinically undetectable until found on screening. Occult bleeding, acute bleeding, or changes in stool are observed in less than 5% of patients with polyps.

Adenomatous or precancerous polyps may differ in their gross appearance (as viewed directly through the lens of the endoscope), microscopic features, and size. Viewed directly, some polyps will appear as a mushroom-like growth, with a stalk and bulb. These polyps are called PEDUNCULATED. Other polyps will appear relatively flat, spreading along the mucosal surface; these are referred to as SESSILE. Polyps are further distinguished by the way in which their cells are organized when viewed under the microscope, classified as TUBULAR, VILLOUS, or mixed TUBULOVILLOUS. Sessile polyps are more likely to be villous and villous adenomas are more likely to transform into cancer. In addition to microscopic cellular characteristics, size also predicts probability of transformation to cancer. A 1-centimeter polyp has only a 1% risk of containing invasive cancer cells, but that risk goes up to 10% for a polyp larger than 2.5 centimeters (1 inch) (Figure 2-1).

The factors that predispose the colonic mucosa to form polyps impact the entire colon. Doctors know this because of two observations: one-third of patients found to have polyps have more than one, and patients with one polyp have a 50% probability of another polyp being found in the future. Related observations and laboratory research suggest that from their initiation, adenomatous polyps require five years to become clinically evident (visible through an endoscope) and five more years to develop invasive cells. Our understanding of the biology of adenomatous polyps has led to a highly stratified set of screening recommendations (to be discussed later in this chapter).

You might expect a discussion of precancerous changes of the colon to seem irrelevant and after the fact to newly diagnosed cancer patients like

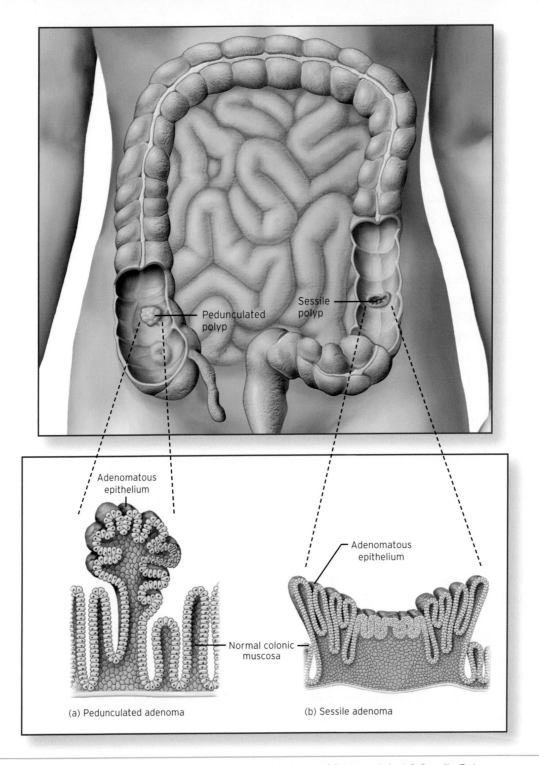

Figure 2-1: Gross Anatomy View Related to Microscopic View of Pedunculated & Sessile Polyp

Doris and Eric, but much to the contrary they listen intently. They need to know how their cancer developed, why there were no earlier clues, why they were not recommended for screening, or why the recommended screening failed to find the polyp in a precancerous state. For patients to begin to invest themselves in the process of healing, they have to reach closure on these ghosts that haunt them. So we will continue as my patients do by reviewing the screening tests, their attributes and limitations, designed to detect precancerous changes of the colon.

Screening for Colon Cancer

The ultimate goal of cancer research is to prevent the disease the way vaccination has eradicated polio and smallpox. In the absence of a definitive prevention strategy, medical science's best efforts have been applied to finding or SCREENING for the disease early enough so that it is virtually curable in 100% of those in whom it is found. There have been unquestioned successes, the PAP SMEAR being the best example, as it permits the early detection and cure of cervix cancer. Some cancer screening tests that attempt to find the cancer early, before it produces symptoms and when it is curable, have had mixed success and remain controversial, like the screening tests for prostate, breast, and lung cancers. It seems not a month goes by without a major news story about a scientific study calling into question the value of PSA screenings or mammograms. The elaborate and often complex scientific studies are reduced to 30-second sound bites that give the impression that we might as well just roll the dice when it comes to the early detection of prostate and breast cancers. Although I appreciate the science and recognize the need to scrutinize both the cost and value of all medical interventions, I remain steadfast in my support of early detection by the best-proven means available, which includes annual mammograms and PSA.

My logic is simple. Cancer evolves from a precancerous state to a noninvasive cancerous state to an invasive cancerous state. The greater the number of cancer cells, the greater the risk of mutation to an invasive state. The greater the number of invasive cells, the greater the risk of those invading cells escaping into the circulation. The greater the number of cells in the circulation, the greater the likelihood that some will anchor and nest in the blood vessels of another organ, creating metastases. The greater the probability of metastases, the lower the probability of cure. Following this logic, the key to success in cancer management is to find cancer before it is invasive, or if invasive, as soon as possible before it METASTASIZES.

Fortunately, there is no controversy in regards to colon cancer screening successfully detecting precancerous polyps and early cancers and most importantly saving lives. The controversy that surrounds colon cancer screening concerns which screening tool is best. An effective screening tool must have both SENSITIVITY and SPECIFICITY. Insensitive tests will miss abnormalities. Sensitive tests that are not specific will reveal abnormalities that are not related to the cancer, often leading to more tests, procedures, and anxiety that may not only be unhelpful but seriously harmful. The most effective screening tool will be the one that is the most sensitive and the most specific. Colonoscopy is clearly the most sensitive and most specific tool. So one might wonder why there is controversy. In a recent survey conducted by the American Cancer Society, only 29% of the 130,000 age-appropriate at-risk U.S. citizens queried about colon cancer screening had undergone age-appropriate colon cancer screening by colonscopy. The controversy is this: We have a highly sensitive and very specific screening tool that is perceived as not very patient friendly and therefore sadly underutilized. In its place an array of less sensitive and less specific screening tests are offered. These tests include: FECAL OCCULT BLOOD TESTING, DOUBLE CONTRAST BARIUM, and SIGMOIDOSCOPY. Relatively new in the potpourri of colonoscopy alternatives is VIRTUAL COLONOSCOPY. Let's begin by reviewing colonoscopy to understand why it remains the gold standard and why these lesser alternatives don't stack up.

Diagnostic Studies

To understand why colonoscopy is the gold standard of colon cancer screening tests we need to return once again to the concept of sensitivity and specificity. The most sensitive and specific screening test for colon cancer would be one that visualizes the entire colon, visualizes it directly, permits biopsies of abnormal areas, has minimal physical risk, and could be performed at reasonable cost. COLONOSCOPY is the only screening test that meets all of these requirements (Figure 2-2).

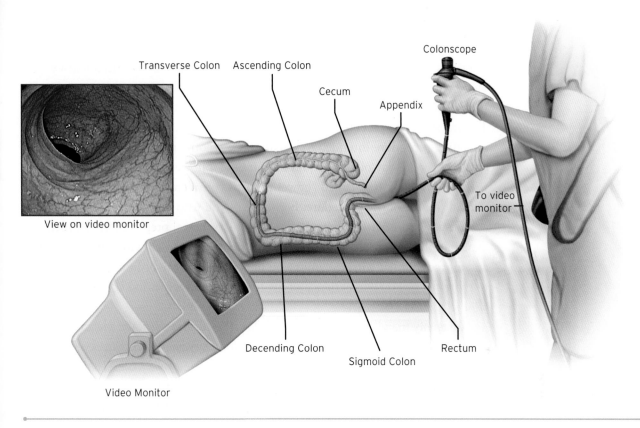

Transverse Colon   Ascending Colon

Cecum

Appendix

Colonscope

To video monitor

View on video monitor

Video Monitor

Decending Colon

Sigmoid Colon

Rectum

Figure 2-2: Colonoscopy

The development of fiberoptic technology permitted the design of flexible endoscopes that can be inserted into body cavities. Such devices are used to evaluate diseases of the stomach, urinary tract, lungs, colon, etc. Beginning 40 years ago these flexible fiberoptic endoscopes replaced rigid metal endoscopes, which had much more limited application. The evolution of industrial polymers and fiberoptic technology permitted the design of flexible hollow tubes, the lumens or channels of which could be subdivided for selected purposes. Each of the four sub channels of a standard endoscope has a designated purpose (picture four drinking straws clustered and bound with black electrical tape): one for a fiberoptic cable to visualize the body cavity; one for insufflation of air, instillation of irrigation fluid, and to suction to clear the path in front of the advancing scope; one for a light to illuminate the path in front of the advancing scope; and one through which wires could be advanced to hook onto and retrieve material of interest as visualized through the fiberoptic camera lens, i.e., obtain a biopsy.

To permit an unimpaired view of the entire colon mucosa the colon must be clear of any fecal matter that might obscure the gastroenterologist's view. Minimal amounts of feces might be irrigated and suctioned away via the COLONOSCOPE but the colon should be 99% empty to maximize viewing. The safest way to prepare a colon for the colonoscopy, or for that matter any screening procedure intended to visualize the colonic mucosa, is to combine a pre-procedure day of clear-liquid-only intake followed by bowel cleansing with laxatives. This so-called "bowel-prep" is considered by many patients the difficult aspect of the procedure. For those of you who may not have had a colonoscopy, alternative screening procedure, or bowel prep, a more detailed explanation is in order. For those of you who are diagnosed with colon cancer and all too familiar with the prep, you may find empathy or humor as I digress to share my personal experience of my first prep and screening colonoscopy.

When my friend, who is a gastroenterologist, explained the bowel preparation or "prep," I was loath to realize I couldn't eat or drink anything other than clear liquids the day before the procedure. "That'll be 36 hours without solid food," I said, stating the obvious. I whined like a child. I pleaded my case that I exercise everyday and couldn't fast that long. He lost patience with me and recommended I skip the exercise for a day. My whining continued until he relented by allowing me to eat Jello the day before the procedure. He laughed saying that once I started the prep I'd have little interest in food anyway; I didn't appreciate the humor of the comment.

A week had passed since I spoke to my gastroenterologist in preparation for my first colonscopy and I had begun the countdown to the procedure day. Three days to go, I read the package insert on the prep. Two days to go, I carb loaded for dinner then made four pans of Jello so they would set overnight. Procedure day minus one, I scheduled no patients after 3 P.M. so I could be home by 5 P.M. to begin the prep. I arrived home before my wife and children returned from work and school. I mixed my prep as directed, 1.5 ounces of Fleet's phosphosoda with 4 ounces of ginger ale. I drank the salty solution in one swallow then finished off the 12-ounce can of ginger ale. I followed it almost immediately with 24 ounces of water. I was probably a bit aggressive with the rapid hydration but I just wanted to get it over. About an hour later my wife arrived home and she inquired how I was feeling knowing I had come home early to take the laxative. Just as I finished saying "I'm fine, nothing has happened yet," I felt the first inner rumblings. I spent the following hour in the bathroom, not uncomfortable, just in dispose. By the end of the second hour on the commode, what was coming out of me looked very much like the water I hydrated with a few hours earlier. In another hour I was to repeat the prep but began considering skipping it. Other colleagues told me they never made it through the second prep and I knew that some patients were successfully cleansed with a single prep. My inner voice reminded me that I had transferred my care to doctors whose instructions I was going to follow.

Convinced that I was adequately cleansed I nonetheless followed instructions and completed the second prep just as I had done the first. Once again it took about 90 minutes for activity but the initial activity was not as clear as it had been. I suddenly found my anxiety turned 180 degrees. Now I was concerned that I wouldn't be prepped adequately enough and there was no way I wanted to go through all this again. I calmed myself by thinking about the science of this process. I'm using a laxative to empty my colon of content but my colon's contents originated in my mouth. So the cleaning process really began 24 hours earlier when I stopped putting food in my mouth. The only things consumed since then were clear liquids, which should transit quickly and not leave residue behind. The first prep cleansed the colon of its contents but not the small intestine. Any residual solid content in the small intestine may still be working its way down to the colon necessitating the second prep. The second prep increased the probability, to better than 95%, of a clean colon that would present a clear view for the GI doctor performing the colonoscopy. Knowledge can occasionally be reassuring; I settled down and soon went off to sleep. The next morning I had the procedure, but as a result of the sedating pre-medication, I have little recollection.

The colonoscopy procedure itself is associated with minimal risk. Patients may experience mild, cramping-type gas pains as a result of the insufflation of air, which is why many gastroenterologists recommend mild sedation during the procedure. To visualize the adequately prepped colon and rectum, a gastroenterologist inserts the colonoscope into the rectum and colon via the anus. The colonoscope is approximately 7 feet long with a gradual contour from origin to end beginning with a diameter about the size of an adult thumb and ending with a diameter the size of a pinky. The narrow end is inserted via the anus and gradually advanced until the entire colon has been traversed then slowly withdrawn. The gastroenterologist advances the narrow end with one hand while holding a docking station in the other hand to which the wider end is connected. The docking station has the camcorder-like camera lens attachment and facilitates the insufflations, irrigation, suction, and biopsy (Figure 2-3).

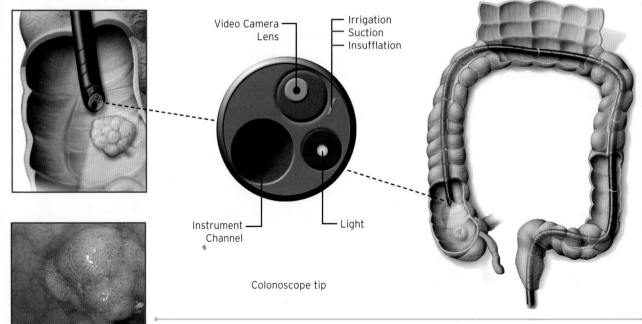

Figure 2-3: Colonoscopy & Colonscope

Virtual and real scope view of pedunculated polyp

If an abnormality is visualized the gastroenterologist will advance one of the wire biopsy devices (picture a piano wire) through the designated channel to sample or biopsy, the abnormality. One piano wire has a pipe cleaner-like brush at its end, which can dislodge cells, which then adhere to the brush; this is called a BRUSH BIOPSY. Another piano wire has a pincer, or forceps, at the end, which can be advanced and manipulated to pinch and tear off a piece of an abnormal area, referred to as a FORCEPS BIOPSY. The forceps remain pinched while the wire is withdrawn so the specimen can be retrieved and sent to a pathologist for review. (Remember that cells are microscopic so it does not take many cells on a brush or a very large pinch to provide a lot of material for the pathologist to review under the microscope.)

If a pedunculated polyp is identified, the gastroenterologist can advance a third type of biopsy wire. This wire has a lasso-like snare at its end, which can snare the polyp, tearing it off at the base of its stalk and in its entirety. Such a procedure is referred to as an ENDOSCOPIC POLYPECTOMY.

Overall, colonoscopy is safe, effective, sensitive, and specific in the prevention of colon cancer. Given the merits of colonoscopy, why do less effective alternatives continue to proliferate? Let's review the alternative screening procedures to see if we can answer this question.

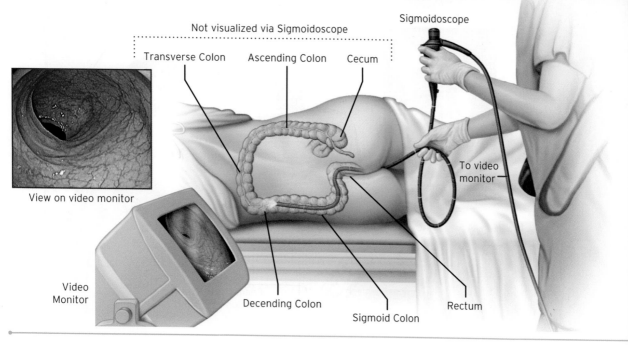

Not visualized via Sigmoidoscope

Transverse Colon   Ascending Colon   Cecum

Sigmoidoscope

View on video monitor

To video monitor

Video Monitor

Decending Colon

Sigmoid Colon

Rectum

Figure 2-4: Sigmoidoscopy

SIGMOIDOSCOPY is quite similar to colonoscopy except that the scope is about one-third the length of the colonoscope (Figure 2-4). The SIGMOIDO-SCOPE is longer than the rigid PROCTOSCOPES that were once the only available tool to directly visualize the mucosa of the distal sigmoid colon and rectum. During the era of rigid endoscopes it was believed that the vast majority of colon cancers arose in the descending and sigmoid colon and rectum, so it was natural to develop the sigmoidoscope for this limited view when the technology became first available. Unfortunately, we now realize that as many as half of all colon cancers arise in the cecum, ascending colon, and transverse colon beyond the reach of the sigmoidoscope, making the limited view inadequate.

The bowel-prep, procedural indignity, risks, and discomfort of the sigmoidos-copy procedure are the same as colonoscopy so the patient is spared none of the distasteful aspects of the procedure. Additionally, this procedure's lesser sensitiv-ity requires a 5-year interval screening rather than the 10-year interval currently recommended after a negative colonoscopy in a low-risk individual. Given the facts, it's hard to understand why screening sigmoidoscopy is still performed.

DOUBLE CONTRAST BARIUM ENEMA (DCBE) represents a non-endoscopic alternative for colon cancer screening. A contrast-containing enema is followed by air insufflation to dilate the colon and distribute the contrast, permitting

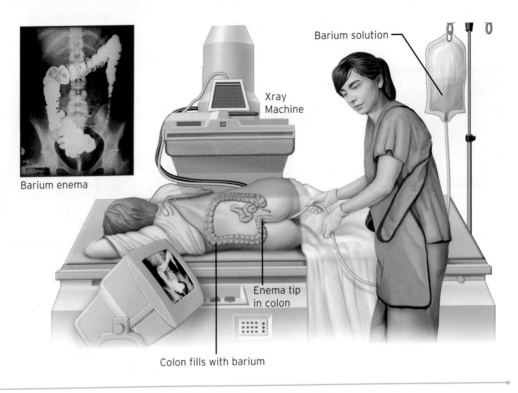

Figure 2-5: Barium Enema Procedure and Radiographic Image

conventional x-ray imaging of the entire colon and rectum. However, should a mucosal abnormality be identified, a colonoscopy will still be needed for both confirmation by direct visualization as well as for biopsy or POLYPECTOMY. Once again the patient is neither spared bowel prep, procedural indignity, nor discomfort as a clearly less sensitive and less specific alternative to colonoscopy is employed. Additionally, like sigmoidoscopy, this procedure's lesser sensitivity requires a 5-year interval screening rather than the 10-year interval currently recommended after a negative colonoscopy in a low-risk individual (Figure 2-5).

VIRTUAL COLONOSCOPY is a recent addition to the list of colonoscopy alternatives. This procedure is similar to the barium enema except that COMPUTERIZED AXIAL TOMOGRAPHY (CT or CAT scan) is used to visualize the colon, rather than conventional x-ray imaging. Although the sensitivity and specificity appears to be greater than with DCBE the same negatives apply to this emerging technology as bowel prep and need for confirmatory colonoscopy are needed. However, there may be a future role for virtual colonoscopy as an initial screening procedure for low-risk individuals. If the entire population were to embrace screening colonoscopy according to current screening guidelines the need for the procedure would certainly outstrip the physician resources available to perform it. There would be a need for screening alternatives that would limit the demand for gastroenterologist-performed colonoscopies, and virtual colonoscopies may fill that void (Figure 2-6).

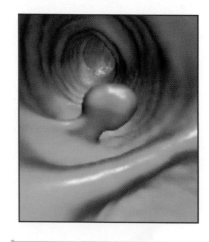

Figure 2-6: Polyp as Viewed by Virtual Colonoscopy

The least invasive of the alternative colon cancer screening procedures involves stool analysis. The association of occult colonic mucosal bleeding with colon polyps led to the obvious conclusion that decomposed blood in the stool, invisible to the unaided eye, might provide a valuable clue to the presence of diseased colonic mucosa. To assess the presence of blood in feces researchers developed biochemical tests called FECAL OCCULT BLOOD TESTS (FOBT). The patient or examining doctor places a fresh sample of stool on a cardboard card and applies a chemical reagent that identifies a component of blood, like iron. If iron is present the chemical reaction between the reagent and the iron stains blue an impregnated disc in the center of the cardboard card. The blue stain confirms the presence of iron, which in turn suggests the presence of blood, which warrants a colonoscopic evaluation.

Although FOBT is easy, more dignified, and less expensive, the test is neither specific nor sensitive. Sensitivity is compromised because precancerous mucosal lesions rarely bleed, and if bleeding is associated with a precancerous lesion or early cancer, that bleeding tends to be intermittent. Specificity is compromised because blood could be in the stool but come from sources unrelated to colon cancer, like gastritis. Additionally, specimen handling, food interference, and medication contamination may also limit the effectiveness of FOBT. The high frequency of both false-positive tests (blood found unrelated to cancer) and false-negative tests (blood not observed despite the presence of a polyp or cancer) make classical FOBT of limited value in the early diagnosis of colon cancer and essentially of no value in screening for precancerous polyps.

However, despite the limitations of FOBT the concept of a non-invasive stool-based screening for colon cancer and precancerous polyps remains attractive and has been proven to decrease colon cancer deaths. It therefore remains a part of the annual physical in conjunction with a DIGITAL RECTAL EXAM OR DRE (Figure 2-7). Recent advances in the understanding of the

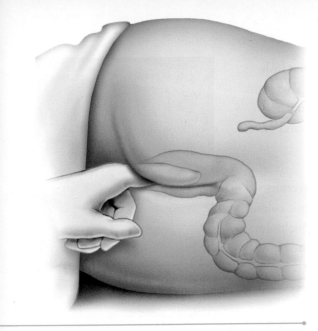

Figure 2-7: Digital Rectal Exam

molecular biology of colon cancer carcinogenesis has led to the development of FECAL DNA TESTING. This is a screening test that detects genetic mutations characteristic of colon cancer in mucosal cells that are shed (like dry skin) in the stool. The advantages over classical FOBT are many: first, only a single stool sample is needed since genetic changes are permanent as opposed to the bleeding which is intermittent; second, there are no diet or medication interferences; third, some genetic changes will precede malignant transformation so in theory DNA testing could screen for pre-malignant adenomas whereas FOBT will likely only detect the bleeding associated with a cancer. Unfortunately, this test is quite expensive, is neither as sensitive nor as specific as colonoscopy, and still requires colonoscopic confirmation of abnormalities.

The general population, those without a family or personal history of colon cancer, adenomatous polyps, or predisposing colon disease are at low risk for colon cancer. Low-risk persons are recommended for colon cancer screening to begin at age 50 and be repeated every 10 years following a normal study. The incidence and the age of onset of colon cancer for African-Americans have prompted a recent recommendation to begin low-risk screening at age 45. The observation of polyps during a screening exam would elevate that individual's risk profile, necessitating more frequent surveillance (Table 2-8).

Doris was among the 10% of patients who, despite following screening guidelines nonetheless developed an invasive cancer of the rectum. Eric, on the other hand was among the 10% of colon cancer patients diagnosed prior to age 50. Was Eric genetically predisposed to colon cancer? Should Eric have been undergoing screening in his 30s? Are there blood tests to aid in the identification of high-risk individuals who may develop colon cancer before age 50? These were Eric's questions. The following discussion of hereditary colon cancer syndromes is how I answered them.

Colorectal Cancer Screening Recommendations for Individuals at Average Risk (asymptomatic patients age 50 years or older, 45 years or older if African ancestry)

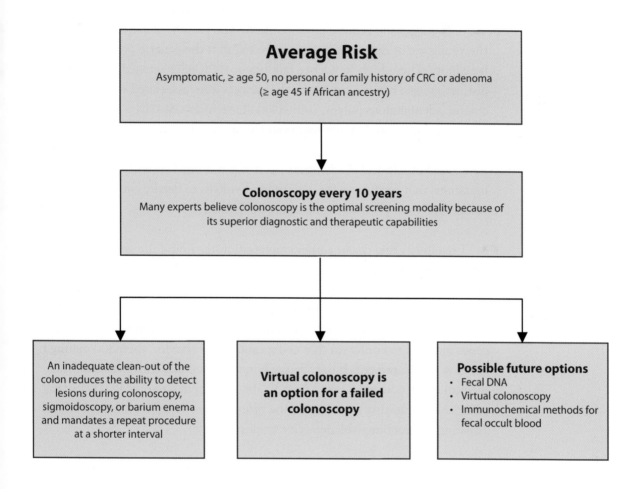

Table 2-8: Colorectal Cancer Screening Recommendations for Average Risk Individuals

Hereditary Colon Cancer and Genetic Testing

Nearly 100 years ago physicians began documenting families with a remarkably high multi-generation incidence of colon cancer, suggesting genetic predisposition. The pattern of cancer incidence and the young age at diagnosis further suggested that the genetic predisposition was hereditary. These high-incidence families or PEDIGREES seemed to fall into two distinct groups: Families in which the cancers were associated with extensive colonic adenomatous polyps, coined FAMILIAL ADENOMATOUS POLYPOSIS SYNDROME (FAP) and families without this association, coined HEREDITARY NON POLYPOSIS COLON CANCER SYNDROME (HNPCC). These original descriptions were based on clinical observations, as it was not until recently that the genetic mutations that predispose the affected individuals to deadly cancers of the colon, rectum, and other organs could be defined.

I reminded Eric of our earlier conversation regarding the genetic basis of cancer: If genetic events govern a cell's behavior, then genetic changes must be present before a cell transforms. However, scientists are still working to understand what changes occur among the thousands of genes in each cell that lead that cell to cancer. If a cell has 30,000 genes and just 1% of those genes mutated to confer on that cell a cancerous behavior, then 300 mutated genes would be present. If only 30 gene mutations could lead to cancer, then medical science would have to find 30 abnormal genes among 30,000 normal ones. Genetic testing for cancer is the ultimate needle in the haystack search. Amazingly, sometimes the detective work pays off.

After many years of scientists searching for the elusive colon cancer genes, the journals *Science* and *Nature*, in 1987, announced the finding of the mutated gene responsible for FAP. The gene was eventually isolated and named APC for ADENOMATOUS POLYPOSIS COLI gene. During this same period researchers were separately working on the specific gene abnormality in HNPCC. Their hard work also paid off as they identified a cluster of DNA repair genes or MMR (MIS-MATCH REPAIR) GENE mutations as the cause of most HNPCC. Today genetic tests for both FAP and HNPCC are commercially available.

FAP is the more serious and fortunately less frequent of the hereditary colon cancer syndromes. The APC mutation, which defines FAP, predisposes to adenomatous polyps. Polyps, in patients with FAP, may be numerous, in the hundreds or thousands and are usually present by the second or third decade of life. Approximately 80% of FAP individuals have a classical mutation of the APC gene. Approximately 60% of newly diagnosed FAP patients will have colon cancer evident on first colonoscopy. All FAP individuals will develop colon cancer before their fourth decade of life if preventative surgery, TOTAL COLECTOMY (the removal of the entire colon), is not performed.

Although cancers in HNPCC individuals also arise in adenomatous polyps, the number of polyps is dramatically less. The classical genetic mutations associated with HNPCC are more varied and are only present in about half the patients who are screened. Regardless of the genetic profile, the majority of patients with HNPCC have a strong family history of adenomatous polyps and/or colon cancer. Up to a third of patients with the hallmark genetic mutations will be the first in their family lineage to have them. Such genetic events are referred to as DE-NOVO ACQUIRED MUTATIONS (Note: Even mutations we consider hereditary have to start somewhere. The de-novo acquired mutation means this is the first generation to have the mutation but all subsequent generations will be at risk). Polyps and subsequent cancer do not usually develop in HNPCC individuals until the third or fourth decade of life. However, polyp transformation is accelerated, necessitating more frequent colonoscopic surveillance and chemoprevention (see Chapter 6). As in FAP, PROPHYLACTIC, elective total colectomy should be discussed with patients with confirmed HNPCC. Female patients with HNPCC who elect total colectomy should as well undergo elective surgical removal of the uterus and ovaries as the HNPCC genetic mutations predispose them to cancers of these organs.

Our increasing understanding of the complexity of the genetic abnormalities associated with colon cancer, and the limitations in routine testing for them, has broadened both the definitions of FAP and HNPCC to encompass clusters of related syndromes. Additionally, a set of clinical criteria has been developed to better define high-risk individuals in whom the readily available genetic tests are equivocal but who have a typical family history and/or clinical presentation. Researchers met in Amsterdam, then later in Bethesda, Maryland, at the National Cancer Institute to develop and revise these criteria—hence the names Amsterdam and Bethesda criteria. The development of genetic tests, as well as clinical criteria help to not only define patient risk and appropriate screening/prevention strategies but also to evaluate at-risk family members.

According to the Amsterdam and Bethesda criteria, genetic testing should be performed on those individuals at high risk for the HNPCC cancer syndromes and include people who have two first-degree relatives (sibling, parent, child) with colorectal cancer or three second- or third-degree relatives with breast, ovarian, uterine, or other specified cancers. There is some suggestion that younger patients (under age 50 years) with colon cancer should be tested even without a significant family history because of their higher chances of carrying the HNPCC genes (possible de novo mutation).

Prevention and screening strategies for persons and family members affected with FAP and HNPCC are complex. For example: The children of individuals with classical FAP (APC mutation) are recommended to begin annual colonoscopy at puberty and undergo elective total colectomy (surgical removal of the entire colon) once polyps emerge. Family members of persons who meet criteria for HNPCC are recommended to begin screening colonoscopy between ages 20 to 25 years, undergo surveillance colonoscopy every two years until age 40, and then annually. As mentioned before, the genetic mutations related to HNPCC also confer increased risk of other cancers especially cancers of the breast, uterus, and ovary, requiring additional screening and prevention strategies (Table 2-9).

Genetic testing and screening guidelines are important because while hereditary colon cancers are believed to account for only 2–5% of all colon cancers, they account for one-third of the colon cancers occurring before age 50, and 20% of colon cancers arise in individuals who do not meet the Amsterdam and Bethesda criteria but have a family history of the disease. These facts suggest hereditary factors distinct from the known hereditary syndromes described in this section. This group of intermediate risk individuals, those with a family history of colon cancer but who do not meet HNPCC criteria (Amsterdam and Bethesda) as well as those under 50, require special attention. Despite medical science's current inability to identify specific genetic mutations in these individuals, an intermediate risk screening strategy has been developed. The presence of colorectal cancer or adenomatous polyps in

Colorectal Cancer Screening Recommendations for Individuals at High Risk

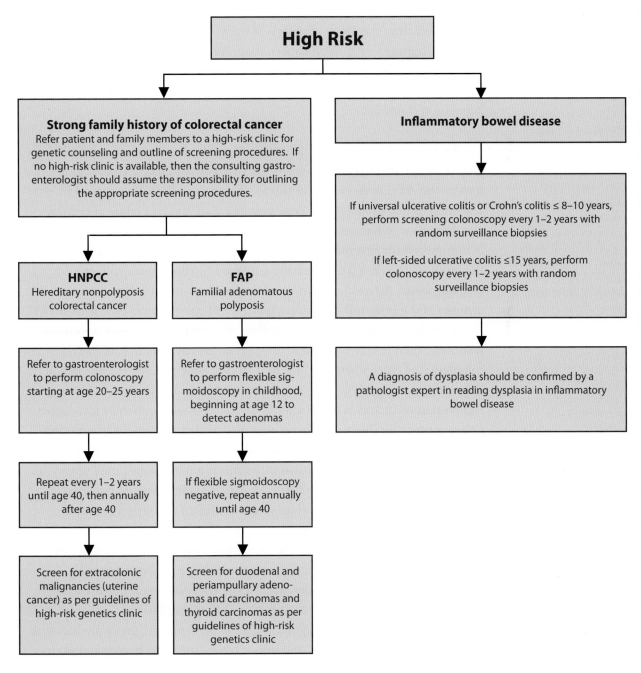

High Risk

Strong family history of colorectal cancer
Refer patient and family members to a high-risk clinic for genetic counseling and outline of screening procedures. If no high-risk clinic is available, then the consulting gastro-enterologist should assume the responsibility for outlining the appropriate screening procedures.

HNPCC
Hereditary nonpolyposis colorectal cancer

FAP
Familial adenomatous polyposis

Refer to gastroenterologist to perform colonoscopy starting at age 20–25 years

Refer to gastroenterologist to perform flexible sig-moidoscopy in childhood, beginning at age 12 to detect adenomas

Repeat every 1–2 years until age 40, then annually after age 40

If flexible sigmoidoscopy negative, repeat annually until age 40

Screen for extracolonic malignancies (uterine cancer) as per guidelines of high-risk genetics clinic

Screen for duodenal and periampullary adeno-mas and carcinomas and thyroid carcinomas as per guidelines of high-risk genetics clinic

Inflammatory bowel disease

If universal ulcerative colitis or Crohn's colitis ≤ 8–10 years, perform screening colonoscopy every 1–2 years with random surveillance biopsies

If left-sided ulcerative colitis ≤15 years, perform colonoscopy every 1–2 years with random surveillance biopsies

A diagnosis of dysplasia should be confirmed by a pathologist expert in reading dysplasia in inflammatory bowel disease

Table 2-9: Colorectal Cancer Screening Recommendations for High-Risk Individuals

a first-degree relative before age 60 or in two or more first-degree relatives at any age warrants early screening. Such screening should begin at age 40 or 10 years earlier than the age at diagnosis of the youngest family member (e.g., your dad was diagnosed with colon cancer at age 49, you would begin screening at age 39). Many experts also agree that such screening should be more intensive, e.g., colonoscopy every 5 years rather than every 10 years as in the low-risk population (Table 2-10).

As discussed in Chapter 1, all cancer is, in the final analysis, a genetic disease. Whether the cancer is the result of classical hereditary mutations such as the APC gene in FAP or the MMR gene in HNPCC or caused by sequential acquired mutations, gene mutations are the root cause of cellular transformation. Changes in a person's genome precede the transformation of normal colonic mucosal crypt cells into an adenocarcinoma. Changes in the proteins, the design of which are governed by those genes, also precede carcinogenesis. A new field of research has evolved to study the sequential changes of the gene and protein composition of colon cancer cells with hopes that a predictive pattern of change will be observed. If such observations are successful, then it may be possible to diagnose an at-risk person before the completion of carcinogenesis. This new field of gene and protein research is called, respectively, GENOMICS and PROTEINOMICS. The analysis of likely gene and protein predictors is called MICROARRAY TESTING. In the not too distant future, we may be able to create a cancer fingerprint or a unique genetic and protein signature or bar code that identifies a cancer in development, before clinical detection and before invasion. In this not too distant future of genomic testing, people found to have a high-risk gene/protein signature might be treated before their cancer develops or be monitored for further mutations.

Routine genetic screening with microarray testing may not be a reality today, but a new type of genetic screening tool may soon be universally adopted in the screening of individuals at risk for colon cancer. It is called MICROSATELLITE INSTABILITY (MSI) testing. Microsatellites are repetitive segments of DNA found throughout the genome. Since the genes predisposing to HNPCC affect DNA repair, and minor DNA damage is happening all the time, the presence of damaged or unstable microsatellites (which are normally quickly repaired) might indicate the type of genetic mutations that predispose to colon and the other HNPCC-related cancers. Such MSI testing is now used

Colorectal Cancer Screening and Surveillance Recommendations for Individuals at Moderate Risk

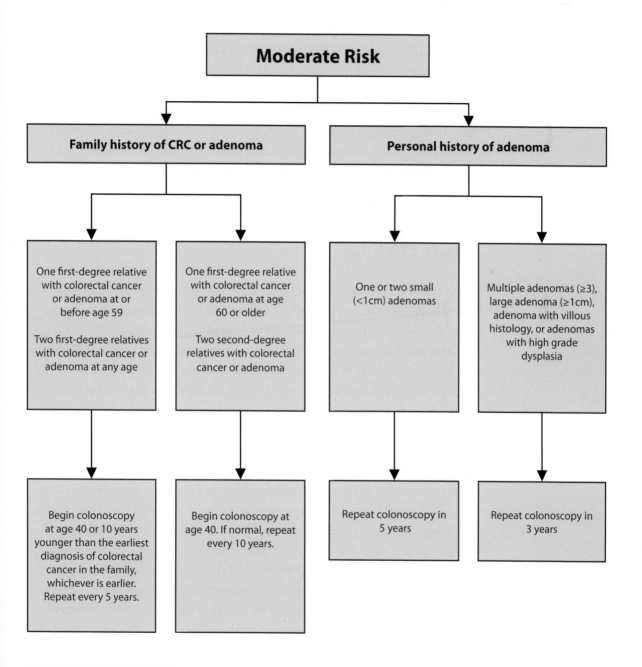

Table 2-10: Colorectal Cancer Screening Recommendations for Moderate-Risk Individuals

to select out those individuals who would benefit from the more specific and more costly MMR gene testing.

Eric did not have a suspicious pedigree to suspect HNPCC. However, his age at diagnosis would raise the specter of hereditary colon cancer. Eric was also worried about his daughter Sarah and decided to have an MSI screening test performed on the surgical specimen and if it was positive to then have HNPCC genetic testing done. Eric and Kim felt like they were starting to catch their breath. Colon cancer was beginning to make sense, but if the cancer was not hereditary then were there any risk factors that could answer the persistent question, "Why me?" for patients like Doris and Eric.

General Risk Factors–Related Diseases–Clinical Findings

Doris and Sam didn't understand how they could do everything right, eat well, exercise, undergo all recommended health maintenance testing including following colon cancer screening guidelines and still end up with Doris being diagnosed with cancer of the rectum. Were there risk factors that Dr. Simon missed? Were there problems with her diet? Was there any way to explain why this happened to her? The simple answer is there is no answer. Sometimes, even when we practice what health experts preach, the cruel hand of fate applies its grip.

Doris's diet was commendable. She was one of the rare people who ate more than five servings of fruits and vegetables a day and on many days she ate no meat at all. I told Doris that the relationship between diet and colon cancer was suggestive but not proven. The lower incidence of colon cancer in countries where people consume most of their calories from vegetables and eat less meat, particularly fried and grilled meats provoked a theory of diet and cancer relationship. The diet theory of colon cancer purports that calcium, plant fiber and plant associated vitamins and minerals are protective against colon cancer; while obesity, excessive calorie intake and diets with a disproportionate percentage of calories from animal meats are stimulatory of polyp formation and their transformation to colon cancer. Unfortunately, no study to date has confirmed these relationships. Sam, who thinks a meal isn't a meal without meat, said, "Thank God."

Inflammatory bowel disease, and prior bowel irradiation like that used to treat cancers of the prostate and cervix, also increase the risk of colorectal cancer, but neither of these applied to Doris.

I explained to Doris and Sam that the only real colon cancer risk factor for the overwhelming majority of people is their age. Cancers of the colon and rectum like most organ cancers increase in frequency as we age. The average age of onset of colon cancer is near 70. Cancer is the consequence of normal cellular aging, and as medicine conquers early deaths from infection and heart disease, our society will be blessed with increasing longevity but at a cost of increasing cancer incidence.

The only other risk factor was Doris's prior history of a colon polyp, but Doris had the polyp removed and followed the surveillance guidelines, initially at a three-year interval then at a five-year interval. How could she have developed cancer with a negative colonoscopy just four years ago? Unfortunately, even when following all the guidelines, 10% of patients develop cancer. Guidelines have helped a great deal to reduce cancer incidence but there is no perfect solution. Doris, like Eric, just happened to be one of the unlucky minority of patients who seem to fall through the cracks.

Doris and Sam decided the glass was half full. They should count their blessings after 50 years of mostly blissful marriage and 70 years of good health. Hopefully the cruel hand of fate just put a speed bump in the road and not a stop sign. Before discussing treatment, they had some final questions that had been echoed by Eric and Kim: "How could this cancer have grown inside me without my knowing it? How could I have had no prior symptoms?"

Signs and Symptoms

As I explained earlier, precancerous adenomatous polyps rarely bleed or produce any symptoms. When symptoms do occur it is usually only after the developing cancer has become invasive. Bleeding is one of the earliest symptoms of invasive colon cancer. It occurs as a growing polyp disturbs the mucosal surface or the pedunculated polyp stalk is torn at its base by passing fecal waste. The bleeding, as discussed earlier, may be acute, demonstrated by a bloody bowel movement or it may be occult, detected in feces by FOBT or by blood analysis after the development of iron deficiency anemia. If the bleeding is coming from the right side or ascending colon and it is heavy, the partially decomposed blood in the toilet may no longer be red but black like liquid tar and is referred to as MELENA. Bleeding, whether directly, in the form of bright red blood or melena, or indirectly, as witnessed by iron deficiency anemia or positive fecal occult blood test, remains the most common presenting symptom.

The second most common symptom of colorectal cancer is change in bowel habits. Cramping or diffuse abdominal pain, CONSTIPATION, and change in stool caliber are most often described. Unfortunately, these symptoms can be vague and intermittent, and as well, are non-specific and associated with many benign conditions. Less often, patients experience rectal pain and abdominal distention, which also are problematic because of their lack of specificity. In the final analysis, the onset of abdominal symptoms or change of bowel habits is ominous as it suggests an advanced cancer that is large enough to compromise normal bowel function.

Fortunately, neither Eric nor Doris had abdominal pain or change in bowel habits, reassuring them that the cancer was in its early stages. There is one last topic to review before patients like Eric and Doris can begin to explore their treatment options: The biopsy. What we can learn from the biopsy procedure and its limitations have a great impact on treatment options.

The Biopsy — Pathologic Evaluation of the Polyp

One of the greatest limitations of the alternative screening procedures as compared to colonoscopy, is the need for a colonoscopy should colon cancer be suspected. The need to confirm the polyp under direct visualization, to simultaneously directly visualize the entire colonic and rectal mucosa for additional abnormalities and to biopsy the polyp to determine its pathologic nature, leave no alternative but to perform a colonoscopy.

A woman or man with a polyp or mucosal defect in the colon or rectum found or confirmed on colonoscopy requires prompt medical attention.

Fortunately, the vast majority of polyps are not cancer. Unfortunately, in most instances, the only way to be sure there is not cancer is to remove some or all of the polyp and view the cells under a microscope. Biopsies range from pieces of tissue no bigger than the head of a pin from a sessile villous polyp, to the

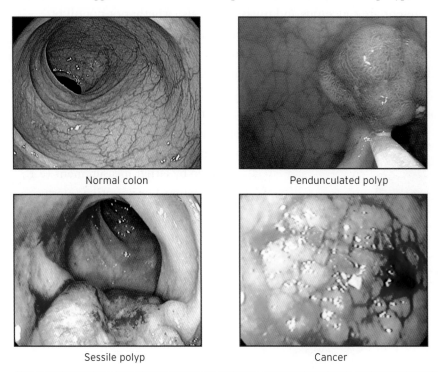

Normal colon

Pendunculated polyp

Sessile polyp

Cancer

Figure 2-11: Scope View of a Normal Colon, a Pendunculated Polyp, a Sessile Polyp, and Cancer

removal of an entire pedunculated tubular polyp. Colonoscopic visualization is used to facilitate the biopsy. The entire procedure is performed in an outpatient environment (Figure 2-11).

Specialized biopsy devices are used to obtain the sample of abnormal tissue extracted through the colonoscope. Either a piece of the defect will be cut out, INCISIONAL BIOPSY (brush or forceps biopsy) or the entire polyp will be removed, EXCISIONAL BIOPSY (polypectomy). Regardless of the technique used, the microscopic or pathologic review will determine whether or not cancer cells are present and whether or not they are confined to the mucosa or invading into the layers below.

Most often, the abnormality is a pedunculated polyp, which the gastroenterologist will attempt to remove in its entirety by performing an excisional biopsy referred to as a polypectomy. The pathologic and microscopic review of a polypectomy specimen must not only determine whether or not the cells present are cancerous and invasive but also whether or not all of the cancer cells have been excised. The only way to know whether or not all of the cancer cells have been removed is to see a halo or rim of normal cells surrounding the entire cancerous area. This halo of normal cells surrounding the diseased cells is referred to as the MARGIN. Margins will be identified as clean (uninvolved with cancer) or dirty (cancer cells extend to the edge of the specimen). A clean margin will be further categorized by the width of the halo by either measurement (e.g., 1-mm margin) or narrative (close margin) (Figure 2-12). In Chapter 3, I further discuss margins as they relate to the final surgical pathology review.

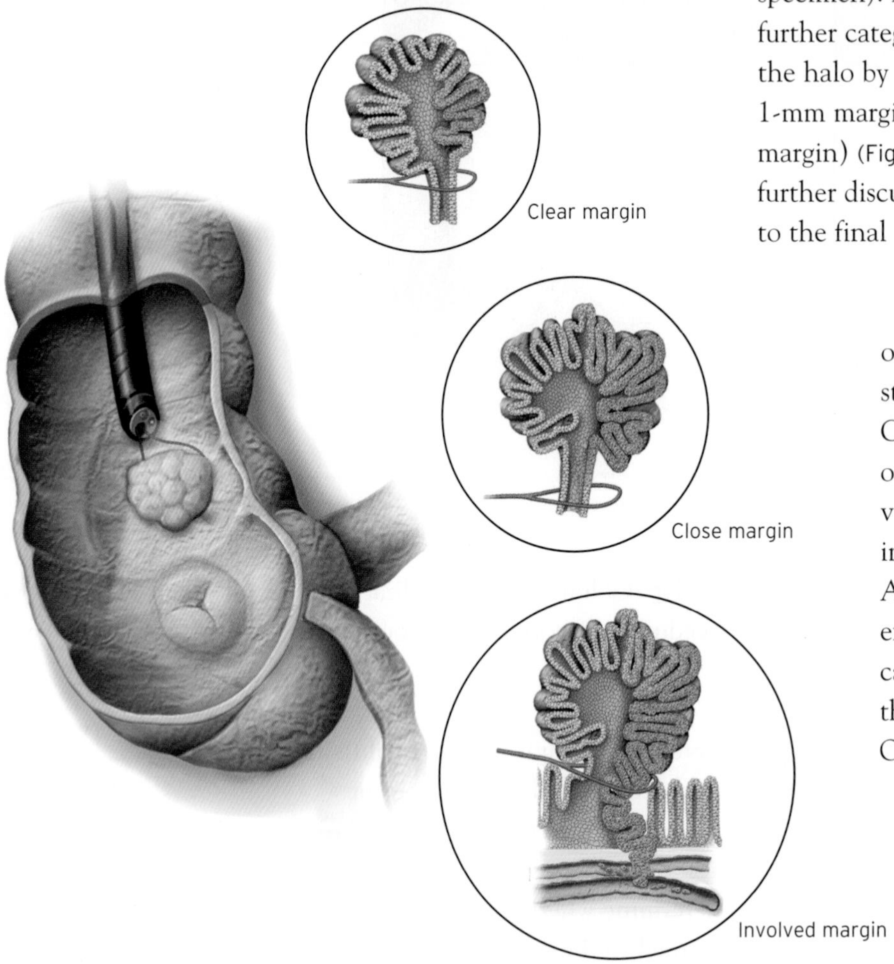

Regardless of the type of biopsy, this is the critical step in defining the cancer. Cancer can be confirmed only by a pathologist's review of an appropriate specimen under a microscope. All of the x-rays, labs, and exams preceding the biopsy can only suggest or raise the suspicion of cancer. Only after a biopsy can the

Clear margin

Close margin

Involved margin

Figure 2-12: Polypectomy margins

pronouncement "you have cancer" be made. After that, all medical efforts are directed at planning the cancer treatment. The finding of invasive cancer adds a layer of complexity to the treatment planning, as we will see in the following chapters.

Both Doris and Eric underwent colonoscopies with biopsy, which in both cases revealed an invasive cancer. In neither case could the cancer be completely removed. In both cases small pieces of the tumor, or incisional biopsies, were performed. The pathologic evaluation would help Doris and Eric, their families, and their doctors select the most appropriate treatment options. Options are both a blessing and a curse, especially when different approaches produce equal results. "Just tell me what I need to do," or "What would you do?" or "What would you recommend to your wife or mother?" are my patients' common refrain. How can patients like Doris and Eric decide upon one treatment option—which they see as a life or death decision—when they feel so overwhelmed and so poorly informed? Doris and Eric had decisions to make, but first they needed to understand that treatment and cure were not just about removing the cancerous colorectal tissue.

Making Sense of
The Treatment

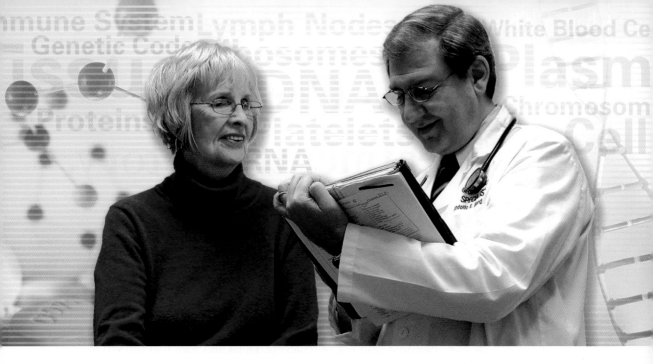

Introduction

This section demystifies cancer treatment planning. We follow along with Doris and Sam as she decides to receive chemotherapy and radiation treatments prior to surgery with hopes of preserving her rectum and avoiding a permanent COLOSTOMY. We follow along with Eric and Kim as I review the surgical pathology and organize the findings into a quantifiable database referred to as STAGING. We review the relationship between stage and probability of cure. We discuss the different types of preoperative and postoperative treatments that can be used to improve the probability of cure. We review how research has improved the outcome for colon cancer patients as well as how ongoing CLINICAL TRIALS allow patients to gain access to new treatments. And we try to make sense of the myriad of measurements used to assess the benefits of these SYSTEMIC interventions. Let's join Eric and Kim and Doris and Sam at their return visits to the office, after the colonoscopic biopsies confirmed invasive cancer.

Chapter Three

Colon Cancer Treatment: History, Science, Practice

Doris had a tumor in the rectum; the area of bleeding was cauterized during the colonoscopy. The tumor was relatively flat, no longer bleeding, and not obstructing. Doris and Sam had time to review treatment options. Doris and Sam understood from their first conversation with Dr. Armstrong that surgery alone would not offer her the best chance of cure, but why? How would radiation and chemotherapy improve upon surgical care? In what sequence would those therapies be administered? And why?

Eric's options were more limited. The cancer was found in his descending colon, near the splenic flexure. The tumor was large, it was bleeding, and it would soon block the flow of fecal waste. Eric needed surgery and needed it soon. Eric and Kim reconciled that surgery was needed now, but they too needed to understand the bigger picture of modern cancer management. They needed to understand the limitations of surgery and what other treatment may follow.

Noninvasive Versus Invasive

Unfortunately, most colorectal cancers that produce rectal bleeding are found when they are no longer confined to the mucosa. They are diagnosed only after there has been invasion into the layers below where blood vessels reside. I had explained to both Eric and Doris that when there is invasion there is a risk that the cancer has not only invaded through the layers of the colon but also through the wall of underlying blood vessels (like the roots of trees growing into pipes below ground), thereby gaining access to the circulation and other organs. One of the greatest challenges of medical science is to develop strategies to find and destroy rogue cancer cells circulating in the bloodstream of the patient with newly diagnosed invasive cancer.

In many patients with invasive cancer, the challenge of finding rogue cancer cells in the circulation is another diagnostic puzzle analogous to finding a needle in a haystack. As you recall from Chapter 1, cells grow by doubling. That rogue cancer cell that survives downstream will become two, these two will become four, etc. Cells are microscopic: 1,000 can fit in a grain of sand, and 25,000 can fit on the head of a pin. None of our current diagnostic tools— neither laboratory tests nor CT, MRI, and PET scans—can detect cancer at that microscopic level. In fact, the only way to detect such a level of contamination is under a microscope (Figure 3-1).

Physicians and patients are in the uncomfortable position of knowing that cancer cells may be loose in the circulation without having any proof. Any observation that might predict the probability of cancer cell contamination

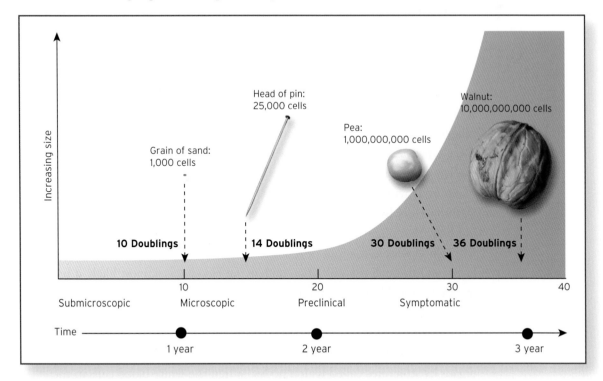

Figure 3-1: Exponential Growth of Cancer Cells

outside the colon is critical to planning the treatment of the colorectal cancer patient. The patient's age, the clinical presentation, and the tumor's depth of penetration into the submucosal layers have all demonstrated predictive value, but the presence of cancer cells within the LYMPH NODES of the diseased area of colon or rectum is the single most important factor in predicting cancer cell spread outside of the colon.

Evaluation Of The Lymph Nodes

I ask patients like Eric and Doris to try to stay focused as I explain the LYMPHATIC SYSTEM and the need to evaluate the lymph nodes draining the area of colon or rectum in which the tumor was found. They need to understand that the presence or absence of lymph node contamination is the single most predictive finding regarding relapse and cure. I begin by explaining the relationship between lymph and blood.

Another type of blood channel runs alongside the blood vessels in the colon and throughout the body. These are called lymph channels. Lymph and blood are related. Blood is composed of RED BLOOD CELLS, WHITE BLOOD CELLS, and PLATELETS, suspended in a fluid called PLASMA. The red blood cells are carrying oxygen to every living cell in the body. The white blood cells are surveying for and destroying foreign invaders (bacteria, viruses, etc.). The platelets are plugging holes in traumatized blood vessels to prevent bleeding. Although all three types of cells circulate in blood vessels, only white blood cells circulate in the lymph system. If we think of the blood as nourishing all of the living cells of our body with oxygen and glucose (sugar), we might think of the lymph as washing every living cell, washing out bacteria, viruses, and anything foreign to our body that might infect or injure it. With lymph channels flowing side by side with blood vessels, if a root or tentacle of tumor has invaded into the submucosal layers and through the wall of an underlying blood vessel, most likely it has also invaded through a lymph channel (Figure 3-2).

Unlike the blood, which flows uninterrupted from organ to organ delivering oxygen and nutrients to each cell it touches, the lymph is filtered between organs by structures called lymph nodes. When the white blood cells in the lymph have surrounded bacteria or viruses, these microbes are filtered out by the lymph node, where special killing cells destroy the foreign invaders, preventing further spread. Unfortunately, cancer cells originate (mutate) from our own cells. Despite their sometime bizarre appearance and aggressive behavior as well as their potential to harm the body, they still appear human to the IMMUNE SYSTEM. Therefore, the cancer cells are not recognized as foreign invaders, and they are not destroyed. They are, however, trapped in the lymph node. If they are living but are trapped, they will multiply, and a nest will grow (Figure 3-3).

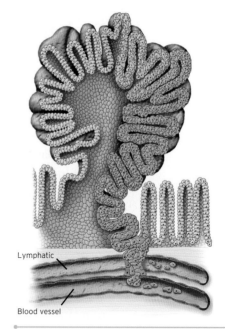

Lymphatic

Blood vessel

Figure 3-2: Invasive Cancer

This is critical knowledge for doctors who are managing colorectal cancer patients. The lymph nodes are a window into the circulatory system and help doctors understand the potential risk for cancer spread. A pinhead-size cluster of cancer cells that would have escaped detection by physical examination, laboratory testing, or radiographic imaging anywhere else in the body can be found in a lymph node when the node is examined under a microscope. If a lymph node is found to be contaminated by a nest of cancer cells, then the cancer likely did not only invade the lymph channel but also the neighboring blood vessel. Lymph involvement confirms that despite removing the cancerous tumor, there may still be microscopic cancer cells contaminating the body. These are referred to as MICROMETASTASES. The relationship between node contamination and risk of micrometastases is linear: The greater the extent of lymph node involvement, the greater the risk of systemic contamination.

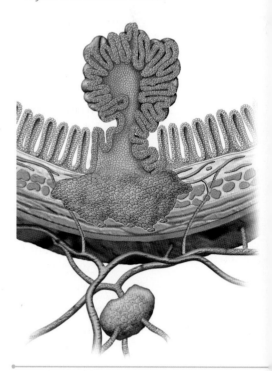

The distinction between noninvasive and invasive cancer, the predictive value of lymph node involvement, and the increasing understanding of the natural history of colon cancer have led to an evolution in doctors' strategies to diagnose and manage a colon compromised by cancer. Having gotten this far with my patients, like Eric and Doris, the next step is to explain the different surgical options. I usually begin this discussion by providing some historical background.

Figure 3-3: Invasive Cancer with Node Metastasis

Evolution Of Colorectal Cancer Management

Despite evidence that the first cancer surgeries were performed in ancient Egypt more than two millennia ago, effective cancer management is relatively new, having its roots in the past century. The greatest obstacles to successful colon and rectal cancer treatments had to do with safe surgical management. Only after Louis Pasteur introduced germ theory, Joseph Lister introduced sterile technique, and Crawford Williamson Long, among others, was able to provide surgical anesthesia, could colorectal cancer surgery become routine. Our understanding of cancer has changed quite a bit over the past century. It was less than 100 years ago that the first effective surgical treatments of colon cancer were published. At that time, surgery was the only cancer treatment, and it was formulated on the notion that cancer was a manifestation of a diseased organ. The only way to eradicate the disease was by radical surgery to remove the entire tumor, if not the entire organ.

At the beginning of the 20th century, doctors believed that cancer would spread from the diseased organ to the draining lymph nodes and only then to other organs. Doctors also believed the size of the tumor predicted node involvement. In 1932, the pathologist, Dr. C.E. Dukes changed the prevailing paradigm by which colorectal cancers had been managed. Dukes observed that two independent factors, depth of tumor penetration into the bowel wall and extent of lymph node involvement, predicted likelihood of METASTATIC cancer spread. He published a system by which colorectal cancers would be assessed for the next 70 years.

By the middle of the 20th century, surgeons were adopting Dukes's theories and establishing the surgical procedures that would define colorectal cancer management for the next 50 years: TOTAL COLECTOMY, RIGHT HEMICOLECTOMY, LEFT HEMICOLECTOMY, SIGMOID COLECTOMY, LOWER ANTERIOR RESECTION, and ABDOMINO-PERINEAL RESECTION. These procedures cover the spectrum from the total surgical removal of a colon or rectum compromised by cancer to a partial removal. After the diseased segment of bowel is surgically removed the remaining bowel is reconnected. The point of connection is referred to as an ANASTOMOSIS, e.g., following the sigmoid colectomy, bowel continence is preserved by a descending colon to rectum or colorectal anastomosis.

If the rectum is completely removed then the remaining colon is connected to a surgical opening made in the anterior abdominal wall called a COLOSTOMY. A colostomy may be permanent, e.g., after an abdomino-perineal resection, or it may be temporary, e.g., to prevent fecal contamination of a colorectal anastomosis during wound healing.

Although the surgical procedures were becoming well defined by the mid-century mark, managing the typical patient who presented with a suspected lower GI bleeding source not visible through the rigid proctoscope was problematic. The first report on flexible colonoscopy was not published until 1967, and this procedure would not be routinely and universally available for another two decades. Computerized tomography or CT scanning was also only in its infancy. Gastrointestinal bleeding during the first three-quarters of the 20th century was evaluated by two relatively insensitive and non-specific tools, the rigid proctoscope and the barium enema. Since three-quarters of colorectal tumors are beyond the reach of the rigid proctoscope, and the barium enema is neither sensitive nor specific, an EXPLORATORY LAPAROTOMY was often required. Exploratory laparotomy is a procedure whereby the abdominal (peritoneal) cavity is opened surgically in order to permit the surgeon to manually inspect the entire length of the small intestine and intra-abdominal colon. For nearly a century, colorectal cancer patients presenting with obstructive symptoms or bleeding underwent these procedures, as they were the best medicine had to offer. Many were cured but there were many who suffered surgical complications, who required permanent colostomies, who relapsed locally, and who developed distant metastases in liver, lung, and bone. *Over the past 30 to 40 years of cancer research, scientists focused on improving diagnostic tools, decreasing surgical* MORBIDITY, *decreasing the frequency of permanent colostomies, decreasing* LOCAL RECURRENCES, *and increasing the percentage of patients cured.*

Basic science research made it apparent that the cancer problem is not what one can see with the unaided eye, not merely a local or even a regional problem of an organ and its draining lymph nodes, but rather colorectal cancer, like all organ cancer, is a total body or systemic disease. The cancer cells gain access to the circulatory system, enabling them to nest microscopically and invisibly anywhere in the body. It became increasingly clear that curing cancer in the 21st century was going to be less related to further refinement in colon and rectum cancer surgery and more related to the ability of medical science to develop treatments that destroy the cancer cells circulating at large in the body or find the cancer before the cells become disseminated.

By the close of the 20th century, barium enemas and exploratory laparotomies had become inconsistent with the emerging technologies available to assess and mange colorectal cancer. Three-dimensional imaging of the abdominal cavity and the organs at risk of metastasis, colonoscopic evaluation of the entire length of the colon and rectum, and endoscopic ultrasound of rectal tumors to preoperatively determine the depth of tumor penetration and node contamination had completely revolutionized the clinical evaluation of the patient with gastrointestinal bleeding of suspected colorectal origin. New technologies like LAPAROSCOPY, a surgical technique that visualizes the intra-abdominal contents through a flexible endoscope inserted via a 1-inch incision had not only replaced the exploratory laparotomy but also introduced a revolution in intra-abdominal surgery. Open surgical procedures, like gallbladder removal or appendectomy, that once required a five- or seven-day hospital stay could be performed laprascopically with an overnight stay. Additionally, this surgical technique allows patients to resume driving and return to work pain free in as little as a week.

By the close of the 20th century the systemic theory of cancer, which stated that lymphatic involvement occurred simultaneously with cancer dissemination via the blood circulation, had necessitated weapons other than surgery in the cancer treatment arsenal. CHEMOTHERAPY, BIOLOGICAL THERAPY, and TARGETED THERAPY emerged as the new systemic weapons that might increase the chance of cure for patients with LOCALIZED CANCER and extend the survival of patients with advanced disease. The QUALITY OF LIFE of the surviving cancer patient had also become an increasing focus of research designed to decrease the morbidity of surgery, to ameliorate the side effects of chemotherapy, and to increase the percentage of rectal cancer patients spared a permanent colostomy. At the dawn of the 21st century, in just over 5 years, between 1999 and 2005, the management of colorectal cancer would change more dramatically than it had in the preceding 100 years.

Understanding the differences between invasive and noninvasive cancer, the emerging systemic theory of cancer, and the explosion of available new technologies helped doctors to both limit the morbidity of colorectal cancer surgery and increase the probability of cure. In the next part of this book we will examine the surgical approaches to colorectal cancer management. I will explain how incorporating scientific theory into clinical practice led to the less morbid laprascopic colectomy; how chemotherapy and radiation treatments are used with rectal cancer surgery; and how medical researchers developed strategies to preserve the rectum, thus sparing rectal cancer patients a permanent colostomy.

Surgical Options In Colon And Rectal Cancer

Many factors should be considered when selecting a surgical treatment for cancer. Physician and patient preferences, patient age and anatomy, tumor characteristics (including size, location, and pathology), clinical presentation (active bleeding, bowel obstruction), genetic profile, as well as patient and family history are all important considerations in how to manage cancer. Doris and Sam were all ears as I began to discuss how all these elements would determine my final recommendations for her cancer management. I suggested we look first at the biopsy findings.

If a polypectomy is performed and reveals carcinomatous changes (CARCINOMA IN SITU or SEVERE DYSPLASIA) but it is confined to the mucosa of the polyp, then removing it, in theory, cures the cancer. However, removal or excision must be complete. To assure complete excision, the pathologist evaluates tissue along the edge or cut MARGIN of the excised polyp to make sure that there is normal colon mucosa surrounding the entire focus of carcinoma in situ.

However, even when all margins are negative and the cancerous polyp has been completely removed, a problem exists: Research has revealed that in other parts of the colon there could be adenomatous polyps or even CIS. If they are missed, diseased areas located in other segments of the colon could emerge later as invasive disease. Therefore, a gastroenterologist must visually inspect the entire colon and rectum mucosa either during the screening colonoscopy or the polypectomy procedure.

In patients with CIS, doctors are not worried about spread throughout the body because as long as the cancer is confined to the mucosa, and an adequate surgical margin is obtained around the CIS, there is no risk of spread through blood or lymph. Therefore, lymph nodes are not removed for pathologic review.

If the polyp is sessile and cannot be completely removed or if the margins of a pedunculated polyp are contaminated then removal of the involved segment of the colon, called a SEGMENTAL COLECTOMY, is required to both remove the entire CIS and confirm the presence or absence of an invasive component. Unfortunately if the segmental colectomy reveals invasive cancer then a definitive cancer surgery would still be required to remove lymph nodes, etc. Since multiple abdominal surgeries increase operative risk, when surgery is needed to remove a polyp, even in the absence of proven invasion in the colonoscopic biopsy specimen, a complete cancer surgery is needed. Therefore, segmental colectomies are rarely performed.

Regardless of the choice of management of the colon or rectum contaminated with CIS, there remains a concern of future cancer risk. Repeat serial colonoscopies are therefore a must. More recently, strategies are being pursued to use medicine to prevent new colon cancers in such situations (discussed later in Chapter 8). When there are concerns about hereditary cancer, molecular and genetic testing can be used to assess and educate those at high risk for colon cancer who may opt to choose preventative, or prophylactic, surgery.

If the biopsy confirms that there is an invasive CARCINOMA, as in Eric's and Doris's cases, the situation is more complicated. The entire segment of colon or rectum and its draining lymph nodes must be removed. The lymph nodes that filter the involved colon segment's lymph circulation may hold clues to the risk that this cancer has gained access to the blood circulation. Those lymph nodes are in the MESENTERY and need to be pathologically inspected. A surgical procedure that only removes the involved area of colon will not be adequate here because the lymph nodes must also be evaluated. The surgical options in a patient with invasive cancer must include node dissection. Research suggests, that a minimum of 12 lymph nodes are needed to adequately assess the risk of lymph contamination. Such extensive lymph dissection can be a challenge for both the surgeon and the pathologist.

Remember the visual image of the intra-abdominal colon as an inverted horseshoe. Keeping that same arc-like semicircle in mind, visualize it now not as a horseshoe but as a hand fan, the kind that might have been used by a geisha. The hinge joint is the vascular origin; the accordion pleated lattice holding the outer fabric to the frame is the mesentery; the outer arc of fabric is the colon. The accompanying illustration helps to capture the concept of the regional divisions of colon, with their respective mesentery, blood circulation, and lymphatic drainage (Figure 3-4).

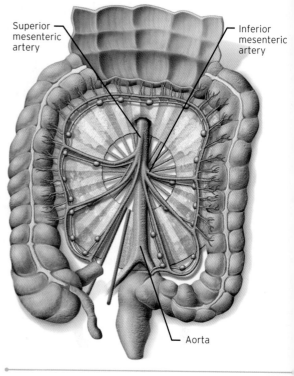

Figure 3-4: Geisha Fan

Although the lymph dissection is an integral part of all colorectal cancer surgery, the specific surgery is determined by the location of the cancerous tumor, as each colon segment has its specific blood and lymph circulation. Tumors originating in the cecum and ascending or right colon are treated with a RIGHT HEMICOLECTOMY. Tumors originating in the descending colon are treated with a LEFT HEMICOLECTOMY. Tumors arising in the transverse colon are managed based on the origin of their blood circulation by either a right or left hemicolectomy. Tumors arising in the sigmoid colon are treated with a SIGMOID COLECTOMY. These surgical procedures are conceptually similar albeit technically very different and are illustrated in the accompanying figure (Figure 3-5 a-h).

As I stated earlier, toward the close of the 20th century it became clear that future refinements in colon surgery were unlikely to enhance cure. It was, however, possible to refine surgery to decrease its morbidity. The first LAPROSCOPIC COLECTOMY report was published in 1991, beginning a new era in colon cancer surgery, which would benefit patients like Eric (Figure 3-6).

Tumors arising in the rectum, such as Doris's present a unique set of challenges to the surgeon intent on removing the tumor and its draining lymph nodes in their entirety, referred to as an EN-BLOC RESECTION. As I explained earlier the goal of the surgery is to remove the entire tumor, the attached mesentery, and the intrinsic lymph nodes such that a clean margin around the tumor is confirmed upon pathologic inspection. There must not only be a clean margin about the tumor both proximally and distally but also circumferentially around the tumor. The rectal tumor not only grows or extends

Before   **After**

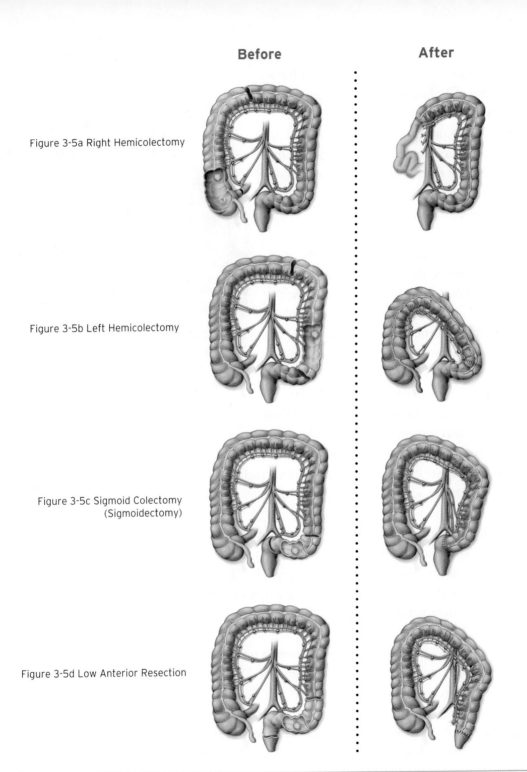

Figure 3-5a Right Hemicolectomy

Figure 3-5b Left Hemicolectomy

Figure 3-5c Sigmoid Colectomy
(Sigmoidectomy)

Figure 3-5d Low Anterior Resection

Figure 3-5a–3-5d: Surgical Options in Colon

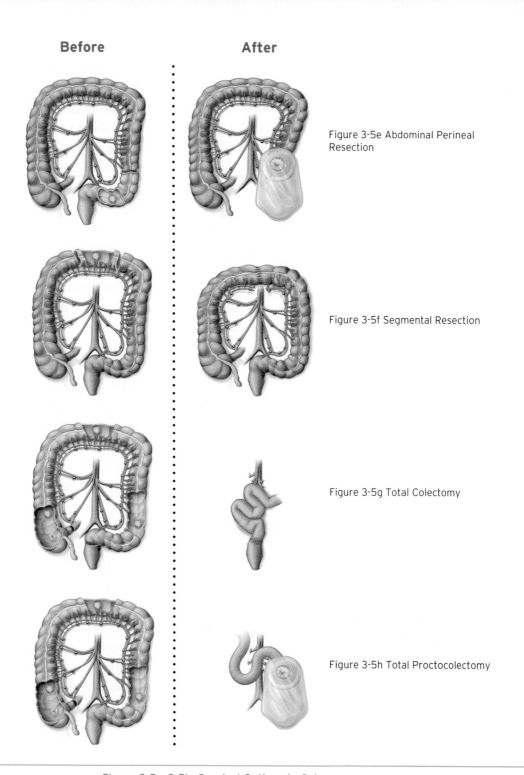

Before   **After**

Figure 3-5e Abdominal Perineal Resection

Figure 3-5f Segmental Resection

Figure 3-5g Total Colectomy

Figure 3-5h Total Proctocolectomy

Figure 3-5e-3-5h: Surgical Options in Colon

proximally toward the sigmoid colon and distally toward the anus, but also it extends circumferentially into and possibly through the bowel wall and into the structures of the pelvis. Obtaining a proximal margin presents minimal challenge as the proximal end of the rectum is attached to the sigmoid colon. Obtaining a distal margin is more complicated as the distal end of the rectum is attached to the anal sphincter and the anus. Disturb or remove the sphincter and stool will leak out constantly (fecal incontinence), necessitating a permanent colostomy. Obtaining an adequate circumferential margin around the entire length of rectum is also tricky as the rectum is anatomically situated in a rather confined vault of bone, i.e., the pelvic cavity. Surgical restrictions within the tight confines of the bony pelvis, the possibility of circumferential growth of tumor into surrounding bone, and the potential for close distal margins as the surgeon tries to preserve the anal sphincter explain why, until recently cancers of the rectum had a five-fold greater risk of local recurrence compared to those arising in the colon.

In the last quarter of the 20th century, rectal cancer research efforts were directed at both preventing the problems of local recurrence and systemic relapse as well as preserving the anal sphincter. Therapeutic radiation was found to be an effective tool that could sterilize the circumferential and distal margins and lymph nodes that were beyond the reach of the surgeon's scalpel. By the time Doris was diagnosed in 2005, radiation had become part of the STANDARD OF CARE in treating nearly all invasive rectal cancers. Radiation not only proved to be effective at reducing local recurrence but also enabled an increasing percentage of patients to be spared a permanent colostomy. Radiation was the next topic for me to discuss with Doris and Sam.

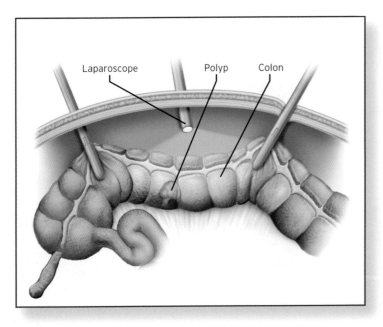

Figure 3-6: Laproscopic Localization of Diseased Segment of Colon

Role of Radiation Therapy in Colorectal Cancer

I explained to Doris and Sam that before they could understand the role radiation would play in her cure, they needed to understand what therapeutic radiation is.

Picture a pebble being tossed into a pond and the wave-like ripples that simultaneously emerge in all directions from the point of impact. Now with that picture in mind, imagine a lit candle afloat in the middle of the pond with its light radiating in all directions. Science refers to that visible light as RADIANT ENERGY (Figure 3-7).

Like the ripples in the water after a pebble toss, radiant energy also emanates in omnidirectional waves from its source, except that these waves are invisible.

Radiant energy is classified by the distance between the waves, referred to as WAVELENGTHS. Wavelengths vary greatly, ranging from wider than a million meters to as narrow as one billionth of a meter. This mind-boggling range of radiant energy wavelengths makes up the ELECTROMAGNETIC SPECTRUM. The shortest wavelengths are those that produce therapeutic radiation. The longest wavelengths are those associated with electricity. In between these extremes, as we move from short to long in the electromagnetic spectrum, are diagnostic x-rays; ultraviolet light; visible light; infrared light; microwaves; radar; and television, radio, and communication frequencies (Figure 3-8).

Therapeutic radiation, also called GAMMA RADIATION, refers to the clinical use of radiant energy emitted by radioactive substances housed in a 2-ton machine called a LINEAR ACCELERATOR.

Like the ultraviolet radiant energy from the sun that can affect skin by damaging cells on the skin surface, gamma radiation can penetrate below the skin, damaging cells internally. Computers and special equipment called COLLUMNATORS permit

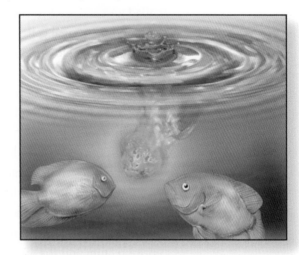

Figure 3-7: Radient Energy

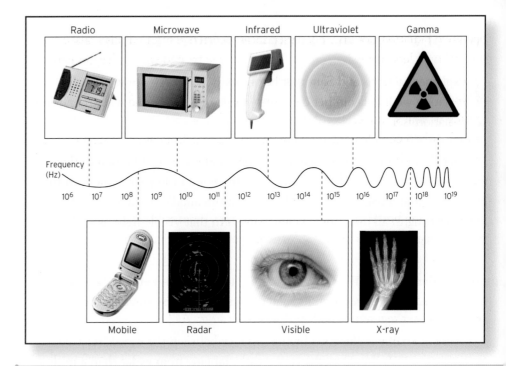

Figure 3-8: Electromagnetic Spectrum

the gamma rays to be focused and contoured to a particular structure of the body like the rectum. At a high enough exposure to gamma radiation, cells may not only be injured but also killed. Research has revealed that there is a narrow range or threshold dose of gamma radiation that when delivered repeatedly (each dose called a FRACTION) to cancer cells, will kill the cancer cells without killing the surrounding normal cells. Therapeutic radiation exploits this research to develop treatment strategies for different cancer problems.

Therapeutic radiation may play a variety of roles in the treatment of colorectal cancer. By the last quarter of the 20th century, unacceptable local recurrence rates after ABDOMINO-PERINEAL RESECTIONS or APR, up to 50% for node-positive tumors, led researchers to evaluate postoperative radiation as a strategy to reduce local failure. Postoperative radiation treatment was proved effective in sterilizing the pelvic cavity of residual microscopic cancer cell contamination after a cancerous rectal tumor has been surgically removed by an abdomino-perineal resection, a surgical procedure which scarifies the entire rectum and the anal sphincter necessitating a permanent colostomy. The success of postoperative radiation led to its use preoperatively. Successful pre operative radiation not only decreased local recurrence rates but also raised the possibility of less aggressive surgery. Rectal tumors treated with radiation may shrink enough to permit conservation of the anal sphincter and preservation of bowel continence in tumors that would otherwise require APR. An organ-sparing or anal sphincter-conserving surgery called a LOW ANTERIOR RESECTION or LAR, when complemented by preoperative pelvic irradiation to sterilize the surrounding pelvic and nodal tissue has proven equal in effectiveness to the more radical abdomino-perineal resection for many patients with rectal cancer.

Preserving bowel continence and avoiding a permanent colostomy[1] without compromising cure has made LAR the procedure of choice for rectal cancer patients for whom this procedure is appropriate. However, even when the entire rectum has been removed via an abdomino-perineal resection surgery, PERIOPERATIVE (PRE OR POST) RADIATION treatments are recommended to prevent cancer recurrence within the pelvic cavity. As I will discuss in Chapter 4, research has also demonstrated that adjuvant 5FU chemotherapy given concurrently with radiation in the perioperative setting not only decreases systemic relapses but also further reduces local recurrences. Today, preoperative concurrent CHEMO-RADIOTHERAPY followed by LAR has emerged as the standard of care for the majority of patients with rectal cancer.

The use of radiation for cancers of the colon is more controversial as the other abdominal organs including the kidney, liver, and small intestine are not very tolerant of radiation. Radiation treatments may also be used to help control symptoms from nests of colorectal cancer cells that may have grown in other parts of the body (metastases), especially in the bone. Novel research in therapeutic radiation is paying dividends as techniques to improve external radiation targeting, to implant radioactive seeds, and to inject targeted radioactive molecules are entering the clinical arsenal.

Doris and Sam now understood why radiation would be needed to treat her rectal cancer, why it would be needed before surgery, why her friend Sylvia, a colon cancer survivor was never recommended radiation treatments and why 5FU chemotherapy would be given simultaneously. Concurrent preoperative chemo-radiotherapy would shrink Doris's tumor, increasing the likelihood that

---

1 In some cases a temporary colostomy is created, until all treatments, radiation, surgery, and chemotherapy are completed.

she would be able to undergo a low anterior resection, have preserved bowel continence, and avoid a permanent colostomy. Sam worried that if radiation was given before the surgery it might sterilize the lymph nodes, making it difficult to know if they were contaminated. I explained to Sam that the colonoscopy and biopsies, the CT scans, the endoscopic ultrasound, and the clinical experience of thousands of patients like Doris provided all the evidence Drs. Armstrong, Drake, and I needed to be confident that the preoperative chemo-radiotherapy approach was the correct course of action for Doris.

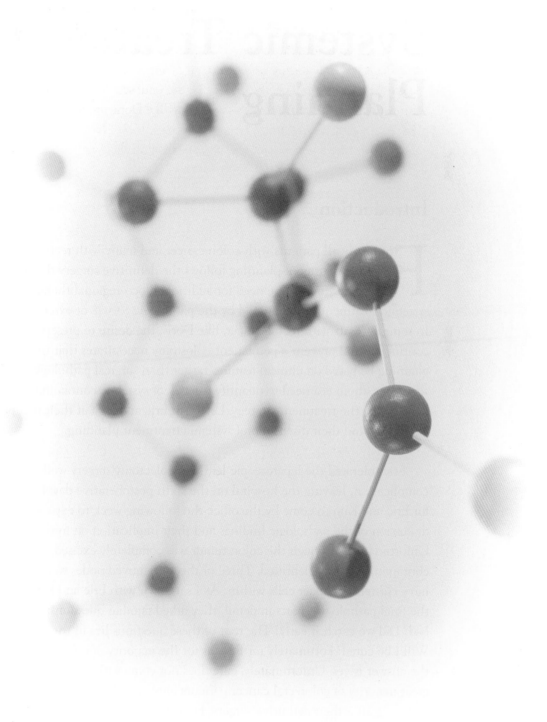

Chapter Four

Systemic Treatment Planning

Introduction

For nearly all patients with colon cancer and many with rectal cancer, systemic treatment planning follows the definitive surgery that removes the bowel tumor. The need for additional loco-regional therapy and/or systemic treatment is determined by the pathologic STAGE or extent of cancer. In some patients with rectal cancer, like Doris, the desire to preserve bowel continence and prevent a permanent colostomy necessitates that treatment planning be based on clinical features rather than surgical pathology. In both situations, there is a need to quantify the risk of systemic contamination prior to selecting the treatment strategy. Let's join Eric and Kim at their first postop office visit and their discussion of systemic treatment planning.

Eric tolerated the laparoscopic left hemicolectomy surgery well, without complication, leaving the hospital on the sixth postoperative day. I arranged for Eric and Kim to come by the office the following week to expand our discussion of the pathologic findings and their implication on further treatment. Unfortunately, although the colon tumor was completely excised, lymph node contamination was identified. Three of the 14 removed nodes were found to have clusters of cancer cells within. As I sat down with Eric and Kim to review the final pathology reports in detail, they asked familiar questions: Is it good or bad? Did we catch it early? The root of these questions lies in the unspoken: Will I be cured? Fortunately for Eric, as for the majority of colon cancer patients, the answer is yes. Unfortunately, cure does not come without a cost, as the great majority of colorectal cancer patients must undergo adjuvant SYSTEMIC THERAPY after their definitive surgery. How doctors determine who should receive systemic therapy is our next topic.

Staging And Grading

For patients like Eric the first postoperative visit comes with much anticipation, as the review of the surgical pathology will determine the probability of cure. The most difficult job I have as an ONCOLOGIST is during this first postop visit when I have to explain to the patient that although the surgeon said, "I got it all," he/she really meant to say "I removed all of the cancer I could see." Microscopic cancer may still be in the body. No matter how positively I try to present the pathology findings, when the probability of cure is not 100%—and it usually is not—a cloud of gloom hangs over the discussion. Eric's chances of cure were excellent but not 100%; so, I placed a box of tissues on my desk and emotionally prepared Eric, Kim, and myself for our discussion.

ONCOLOGY in its essence is a discipline of medical science. In a scientific discipline, theory is tested by experiment, and success is measured quantitatively. In order to quantify the probability of cure or, inversely, the risk of cancer relapse, the oncologist must weigh the evidence that is available. The evidence is to be found in the pathology reports, laboratory tests, and imaging studies, but it must be organized in a meaningful and comparative way. The oncologic medical community responded to this need by standardizing a system for quantifying cancer, both the extent of disease and the characteristics that determine the risk of relapse and the probability of cure. Although it is the physician's desire to comfort and provide hope, there is no escaping an objective review of data with a patient and his/her family before they can provide an INFORMED CONSENT to undergo treatment.

Information gathered about the colon or rectum tumor, the lymph nodes, the radiographic imaging, and the laboratory data comprise the database. The database is organized to quantify or grade[2] the amount of disease locally within the colon or rectum, regionally within the lymph nodes, and systemically within other organs. This system of cancer measurement is referred to as cancer STAGING and addresses each area of disease as follows: the colon or rectum malignant growth or tumor (tumor = T) regarding its size, extent, and location (graded 1 to 4); the lymph nodes (nodes = N) regarding number, character, and location (graded 0 to 3); and evidence of other organ spread or metastases (metastases = M), either there is or there is not (graded 1 or 0). This is called the TNM STAGING SYSTEM. The very least amount of invasive cancer would be represented by

---

2 The word grade also has a technical definition
that is addressed at the conclusion of the section.

a very shallow tumor (T1), without lymph node involvement (N0), and without spread to other organs (M0), or (T1 N0 M0). The worst scenario would be any cancer that had already spread to other organs of the body (T-any, N-any, M1).

Staging allows doctors to categorize patients with similar cancer characteristics, thereby helping to predict outcomes and permit treatment stratification based on risk (Figure 4-1 a-d, 4-2 a-c). Stage I cancers are very shallow (remain localized to the mucosa) and have no proven spread to lymph nodes or other sites. Cancers that penetrate into the muscularis or involve regional lymph nodes are grouped into stages II and III. Any cancer that has spread to another part of the body (e.g., lung, liver, bone) is stage IV. Older staging systems like that published by Dr. C.E. Dukes, are occasionally encountered. These older staging models employ an A, B, C, D system as opposed to the stage I, II, III, IV used in the international TNM classification. (Table 3–5 provides a useful comparison).

Stage Grouping				
AJCC/UICC				Dukes*
Stage 0	Tis	N0	M0	–
Stage I	T1	N0	M0	A
	T2	N0	M0	–
Stage II	T3	N0	M0	B
	T4	N0	M0	–
Stage III	Any T	N1	M0	C
	Any T	N2	M0	–
Stage IV	Any T	Any N	M1	–

Table 3-5: *Dukes B is a composite of better (T3 N0 M0) and worse (T4 N0 M0) prognostic groups, as is Dukes C (Any TN1 M0 and Any T N2 M0)

Doctors determine how aggressively to treat and manage an individual patient based on how advanced the cancer is locally in the colon and regionally in the lymph nodes. The greater the risk of microscopic cancer cell contamination throughout the body (MICROMETASTASIS), the greater the need for treatment to destroy these undetectable cancer cells. This treatment is called ADJUVANT THERAPY because it is most often added to or administered after

Polyp
Bulb-like growth that forms on the mucosal surface.
This tumor may be benign or malignant (cancerous).

Early Stage Cancer
The tumor is confined to the mucosa.

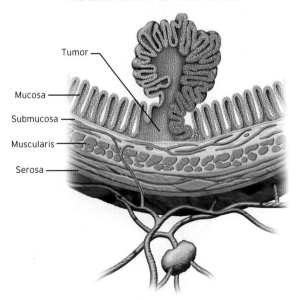

Polyp

Stalk

Tumor

Mucosa

Submucosa

Muscularis

Serosa

Blood vessel

Lymphatic vessel

Lymph node

Stage 0 (CIS)

Stage I $T_1N_0M_0$

Locally Advanced Cancer
The tumor penetrates the muscularis or the
serosa. There is no lymph node involvement.

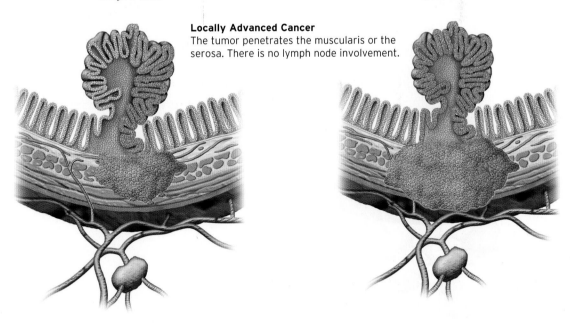

Stage IIA $T_2N_0M_0$

Stage IIB $T_3N_0M_0$

Figure 4-1 a-d: TNM Staging System

Advanced cancer
The tumor has spread to the regional lymph nodes. The tumor may or may not have penetrated the serosa.

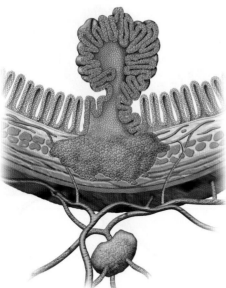

Stage IIIA $T_2N_1M_0$

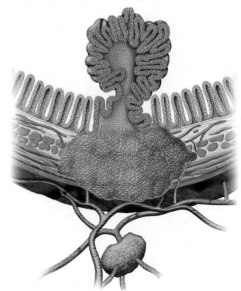

Stage IIIB $T_3N_1M_0$

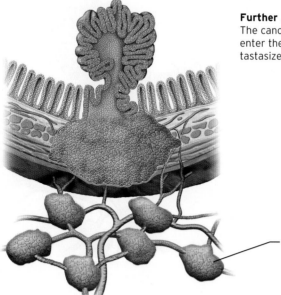

Further Advancing Cancer
The cancer spreads to regional lymph nodes, and/or may enter the blood stream. The cancer can then spread (metastasize) to other parts of the body.

— Lymph node metastasis

Stage IIIC $T_3N_2M_0$

Figure 4-2 a-c: TNM Staging System

the surgery. Cancers proven upon initial evaluation to have spread to other organs (stage IV or metastatic) represent the greatest management challenge. Treatment of such cancers is referred to as METASTATIC THERAPY.

Our evolving understanding of the biology of cancer necessitates continuous revisions to the staging criteria. Subcategories have been added to provide more definition like T4a, b and Stage III a, b, c. Despite these ongoing revisions, a gap will always exist between scientific discovery and accepted policy. The clinical and pathologic findings that fall outside of formal staging criteria but have an impact on patient outcome and the ability to predict risk of RECURRENCE are referred to as PROGNOSTIC CRITERIA. These clinical and pathologic features are further categorized as favorable or unfavorable.

Prognostic features are generally less predictive of outcome than stage and do not always stand the test of time. Some tests like FLOW CYTOMETRY for S-PHASE and PLOIDY (ANEOPLOID, DIPLOID—measures of DNA instability) were once commonplace but are falling out of favor. Others like the postoperative level of CEA (CARCINO-EMBRYONIC ANTIGEN) or tumor-related SEROSAL PERFORATION and BOWEL OBSTRUCTION, have become routine and are discussed later in this book as we turn our attention to specific colon cancer treatments.

The microscopic appearance of the cancer cells has also been used as a prognostic factor. This is referred to as NUCLEAR GRADE and HISTOLOGIC GRADE. A cancer cell that retains it normal cellular and nuclear features is referred to as well differentiated or grade 1. A cancer cell that retains no defining features is referred to as undifferentiated or grade 4. Grade 2 is for moderately differentiated cells, and grade 3 refers to poorly differentiated cells. Like S-phase and ploidy, both histologic and nuclear grade are also falling out of favor as more objective and specific DNA markers replace them.

I explained to Eric and Kim that Eric's tumor had not penetrated through the muscle layer (T2), but the contaminated nodes (N1) resulted in his final stage of colon cancer being a stage IIIa. Additionally, the tumor did not perforate the serosal surface or obstruct the bowel lumen, which is favorable. In its entirety, the staging and prognostic criteria predicted that Eric had a 76% chance of being cured by his surgery or a 24% chance that he would have a relapse and die of this cancer during the next five years.

Eric and Kim were not comforted that the odds of cure were in Eric's corner. They wanted nothing less than a 100% guarantee of cure. I explained that this was not possible, but we could reduce the risk of a relapse by nearly half with adjuvant systemic therapy. We sat down for a lengthy discussion of the systemic treatment of cancer.

Systemic Therapy

The systemic theory of cancer argues that cancer is a cellular disease originating in an organ but possibly disseminated throughout the body at the time of diagnosis. If the cancer were disseminated at the time of diagnosis, then loco-regional treatments would not be adequate by themselves. Systemic or total body therapies would be needed to treat the entire body in order to destroy any undetectable microscopic contaminating disease (micrometastases) or proven cancer spread (metastases).

Efforts to seek and destroy the undetectable rogue cancer cells in the circulation, or the cancer cells nesting in proven metastatic deposits, have led to the development of an arsenal of weapons—medicines that travel in the blood, poisoning cancer cells wherever they nest. Eric asked how these medicines could cripple or destroy cancer cells. I explained how scientists examined cellular structure and function to find ways to disrupt the cancer cells' machinery.

To look at a cell in a scientific way, we would place it under a microscope. There we would see an outer cell membrane surrounding a gelatinous cytoplasm containing a nucleus at its core. Picture the Tootsie Roll Pop, as described earlier, where the wrapper is the cell membrane, the candy is the cytoplasm, and the Tootsie Roll is the nucleus. Within the nucleus is the genetic material or DNA. The DNA is a coded information system like a blueprint or an operating code (software of the cell). For a cell to live, it must continuously uncode DNA messages. Those messages are the blueprint for the production of proteins, the cells' vital machinery. Additionally, for a cell to divide and become two cells, the DNA has to be copied so that the mother cell can divide into two identical daughter cells. An effective systemic therapy would need to interfere with the DNA messages that govern cell repair, growth, and division (Figure 4-3).

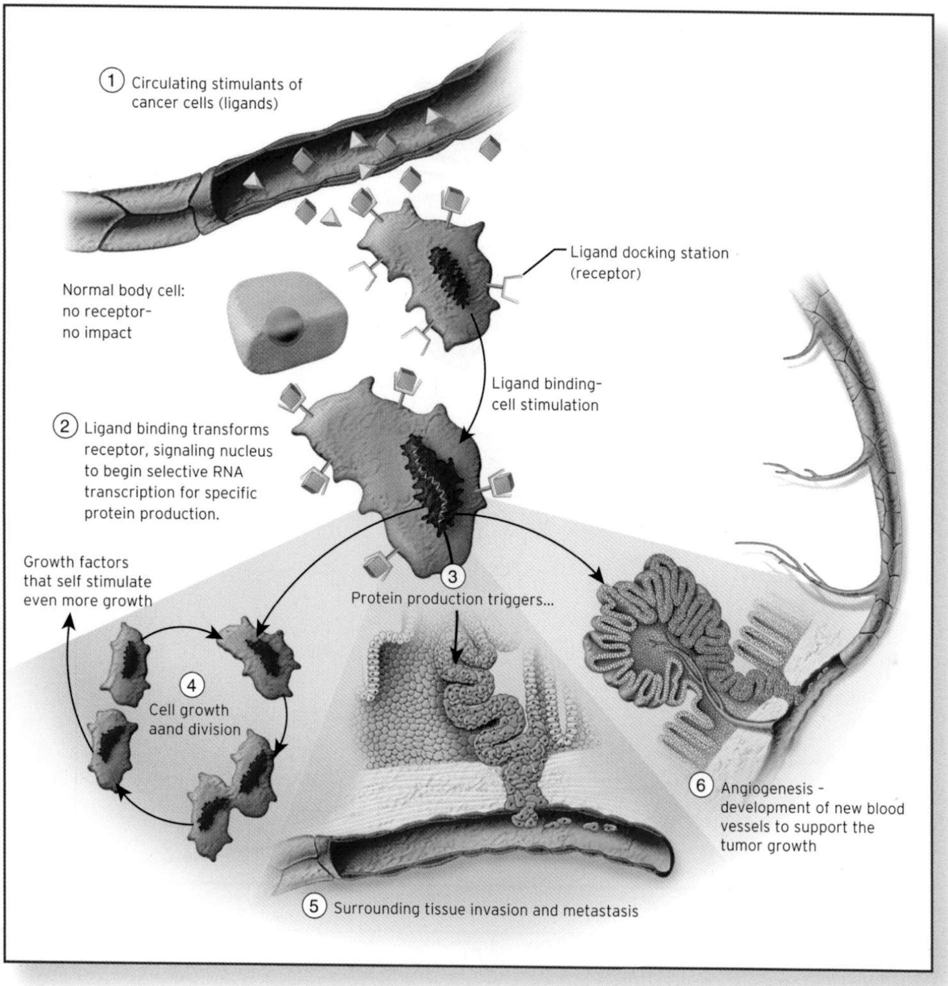

1 Circulating stimulants of cancer cells (ligands)
Ligand docking station (receptor)
Normal body cell: no receptor- no impact
Ligand binding- cell stimulation
2 Ligand binding transforms receptor, signaling nucleus to begin selective RNA transcription for specific protein production.
Growth factors that self stimulate even more growth
3 Protein production triggers...
4 Cell growth aand division
6 Angiogenesis - development of new blood vessels to support the tumor growth
5 Surrounding tissue invasion and metastasis

Figure 4-3: Basic Model of Systemic Therapy

The very earliest forms of systemic therapy were chemicals developed to disrupt or poison DNA. The chemical agents first approved for the systemic treatment of cancer were called CHEMOTHERAPY. The logic of chemotherapy was straightforward. If cancer cells were dividing, they would have to copy their DNA to reproduce. If a treatment disrupted the DNA, the cells could not divide and could not produce daughter cells. Without daughter cells, the cancer could not grow. Furthermore, if the DNA was disrupted, the messages for the production of proteins, the cell's vital machinery that allow the cell to eat, breathe, and remove waste, could not be uncoded. If the cell could not operate its intracellular machinery, the cancer cell would die. Thus, in theory, chemotherapy could stop the cancer growth and kill the cancer cells.

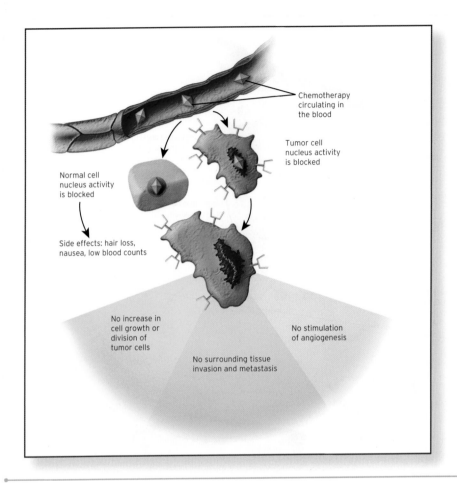

Figure 4-4: How Chemotherapy Works

Unfortunately, like cancer cells, all cells have DNA, and many cells in the body are also constantly growing and dividing: the hair cells, the blood cells, the cells that line the mouth and the intestinal tract, etc. Therefore, these DNA-disrupting drugs were also very toxic to normal cells (Figure 4-4).

Over the past three decades, great strides have been made to increase the effectiveness and decrease the toxicity of chemotherapy. Despite these improvements, both patients and physicians have demanded therapies that are safer, less toxic, and more cancer-cell specific. There was a call for "smart bombs" or "magic bullets" that could seek and destroy cancer cells without harm to the normal cell counterpart. These emerging new weapons in the arsenal against cancer have been called TARGETED THERAPY.

A cancer-specific treatment would by definition affect only cancer cells. However, these cancer cells are so genetically similar to normal cells that they escaped the recognition of the immune system. How could science accomplish what nature failed to do—target the cancer cells? The answer is in the DNA. In the past few decades, through ongoing work to translate the human genome (the basic DNA blueprint of all human cells), scientists are beginning to gain a deeper understanding of what makes a cancer cell behave the way it does. With these insights, cancer management is evolving. Cancer is no longer considered an organ disease or even a cellular one. Today, cancer is considered a genetic and molecular disease. Reflecting these changes, the therapy of cancer today is not just of a cellular nature, but also one of a genetic and molecular nature.

Researchers now understand that within a given cell there are thousands of active genes (specific DNA codes) that define the cell's identity and function. These thousands of genes represent the codes for the thousands of proteins (molecules) that define the cell's structure and behavior. There may be only 1% of those genes, 1% of those important messages that go wrong or mutate, transforming a normal cell into a cancer cell. These mutations result in the overproduction or underproduction of critical proteins that control a cell's growth and behavior and cause that cell to become malignant or cancerous. If researchers could find the 1% of those messages that are mutated, they could then target them specifically and create a magic bullet of cancer therapy. Doctors would then have a treatment that would be targeted only to the machinery gone awry in the cancer cell.

Targeted therapy may sound far-fetched, but history tells us otherwise. Antibiotics were the medical magic bullets of the last century, the targeted therapy of infectious diseases. For many centuries, infection was the leading cause of death in our society. Scientists began to develop treatments for infections by first understanding the molecular differences between bacterial cells and human cells. They were then able to target specific molecules unique to the bacteria, which in turn killed the bacteria and cured the infection without harming the cells of the human host.

As it turns out, targeted therapies for cancer have been around for some time. Observations of breast cancer remission after surgical removal of the ovaries were first reported over a century ago, revealing the relationship between

ESTROGEN and breast cancer. Although sensitivity to estrogen is not unique to the mammary tissue of the breast, estrogen proved to be a powerful stimulant of some breast cancer cells. Antiestrogen therapy, like removing the ovaries surgically or taking antiestrogen pills, proved to be an effective weapon in the treatment of breast cancer while having minimal or modest effects on other normal cells of the body. This type of HORMONAL THERAPY, which has been in existence for over 40 years, was the first targeted molecular therapy. Today, hormonal therapies remain important components in the arsenal of treatments for breast and prostate cancers. HORMONES, like estrogen and testosterone can adhere to the surface of sensitive cells, like those of a breast or prostate cancer, triggering the DNA within the cancer cell to turn on and direct the manufacture of proteins that promote cell growth and division. The circulating hormone is referred to as a LIGAND and the structure that it adheres to on the cell membrane is referred to as a RECEPTOR. Interference with the ligand or receptor, e.g., an anti-estrogen pill, can down regulate the DNA of the cancer cell and in some cases cause cancer cell death.

Although doctors have known about the estrogen relationship to breast cancer for a century, have used antitestosterone therapy for prostate cancer for nearly 50 years, and have been able to test cancer cells routinely for the presence of hormone receptors for over two decades, other molecular targets have, until recently, been much more difficult to define. Today, over 400 molecular and genetic targets and their respective interference therapies are being investigated. The targets include the receptors (found or EXPRESSED) on the cell surface, the ligands that bind to and activate them, the particular DNA that is stimulated by the activated receptor, the RNA translation of the DNA, the proteins which the RNA define, etc. (Figure 4-5).

Thus far, the investigation of two targets, EPIDERMAL GROWTH FACTOR (EGF) and VASCULAR ENDOTHELIAL GROWTH FACTOR (VEGF) has resulted in targeted therapies that have been approved for colon cancer. In both cases the growth factor (EGF and VEGF) and its respective receptor (EGFR and VEGFR) have been successfully targeted. Researchers are investigating multiple agents that interfere with these targets, but only three have thus far completed phase 3 testing and been approved by the FDA. BEVACUZIMAB, also called AVASTIN, is a VEGF inhibitor and is indicated for the first- or second-line treatment of metastatic colorectal cancer in combination with intravenous 5-fluorouracil

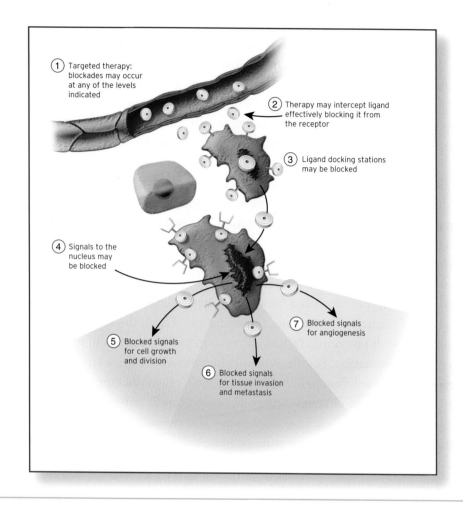

Figure 4-5: How Targeted Therapy Works

based chemotherapy. CETUXIMAB, also called ERBITUX, is an EGF receptor (EGFR) inhibitor and is indicated for the treatment of EGFR-expressing metastatic colorectal cancer in combination with irinotecan (a chemotherapeutic drug) in patients who are refractory to irinotecan-based chemotherapy or as monotherapy in patients who are intolerant to irinotecan-based chemotherapy. PANITUMIMAB, also called VECTIBIX is also an EGFR inhibitor and (panitumumab) is indicated for the treatment of EGFR-expressing, metastatic colorectal carcinoma with disease progression on or following fluoropyrimidine-, oxaliplatin-, and irinotecan-containing chemotherapy regimens. Unlike the antibiotics used to kill bacteria, targeted therapies do have side effects that are significant albeit very different from traditional chemotherapy.

Today not only do doctors need to understand the tumor growth characteristics, the node status, and whether or not there is any evidence of spread to other organs of the body, but also they may need to know if the tumor makes or expresses specific ligands and receptors, e.g., ESTROGEN RECEPTOR expression on breast cancer cells or EGFR expression on colon cancer cells. All of these features have an impact on the local, regional, and systemic therapies that are recommended.

Eric and Kim were becoming anxious knowing that I was about to begin the discussion of Eric's specific treatment recommendation: The type of chemotherapy, the schedule of drug administration, the side effects, etc. I suggested a deep breath and counting to 10 as I took a moment to summarize what had been discussed so far. First, our understanding of cancer has evolved from the disease of an organ to a systemic cellular disease to a genetic and molecular disease. Second, there is a need for adjuvant systemic therapies in patients who are at risk of microscopic systemic contamination. Third, the staging system in conjunction with prognostic factors allows us to predict the risk of microscopic systemic contamination. Fourth, systemic therapies are of three types: hormonal therapy (for selected, hormone-sensitive cancers), chemotherapy, and the newest type of treatment, targeted therapy. For colon cancer patients like Eric who are two weeks out from a left hemicolectomy and patients like Doris with newly diagnosed rectal cancer, there is still one more thing to discuss: How oncologists select and integrate these treatments.

Current Treatment Of Colon And Rectal Cancer

The discussion to this point has focused on the basic biology of colorectal cancer. These concepts apply to Eric, Doris, and all of my patients with cancers of the colon and rectum. Their educational paths diverge now that we begin to discuss patient-specific treatment, as the location of the tumor, its depth of penetration, the clinical presentation, the medical history, etc., will influence each individual patient's management. We will begin with my discussion with Eric and Kim.

Eric and Kim remained anxious as I started to review the standard treatment for a stage III colon cancer with three involved lymph nodes. When I said that there might be treatment options, they groaned. I went on to explain that some of the possible treatments are considered standard, whereas others would require participation in a clinical trial. Their eyes started to glaze over. I decided some background on how a standard treatment is established and what a clinical trial is might provide a better context to understand the treatment options.

For any systemic treatment to become a standard of care it must complete a long and complicated evaluation. The evaluation process incorporates three specific phases of testing: the treatment must first be proven safe PHASE 1, then effective PHASE 2, and then better than the current standard of care that it is replacing PHASE 3. Remarkably, this process can take up to 12 years for each specific treatment under evaluation. Just as the surgical approach to the management of locoregional disease progressed over the past 30 years from the exploratory laparotomy to the laprascopic hemicolectomy, so too has the systemic management of colon cancer evolved. This evolution occurred on two related fronts: the development of effective treatments for proven metastases and the use of those active treatments in the adjuvant setting. Effective metastatic treatments are those that reduce symptoms and prolong the life of patients with advanced cancer. Effective adjuvant treatments are those that reduce the relative risk of cancer recurrence or more simply increase the probability of cure.

The beginning of this scientific systemic treatment evolution can be found in the laboratory research of the late 1940s, which confirmed that certain chemicals could kill cancer cells. A decade later, in 1957, 5-FLUOROURACIL (5FU), one of the first chemotherapy drugs to be discovered, was administered to patients with metastatic colon cancer. By 1968, 5FU chemotherapy treatment of patients with metastatic colon cancer was reported in a peer reviewed journal. More importantly, the first reports of surgical adjuvant chemotherapy were published. Surgeons united to advance the science of cancer treatment, leading to the formation of one of the largest and most successful cooperative research organizations, the National Surgical Adjuvant Breast and Bowel Project (NSABP).

In the three decades between 1970 and 2000, we learned a great deal about the biology of colon cancer but this knowledge did not translate into meaningful clinical improvements. The NSAPB conducted the C-01 trial, which proved that 5FU adjuvant treatment was better than best supportive care. Researchers tested hypotheses to increase the effectiveness of 5FU by giving it continuously;

giving it with the immunomodilatory drug LEVAMISOLE; and giving it with a VITAMIN, FOLINIC ACID (LEUCOVORIN). Despite hundreds of clinical trials and tens of new chemotherapy drugs that were having impact in breast cancer, lung cancer, lymphoma, etc., none of these new chemotherapy drugs by themselves or in combination with 5FU improved colorectal cancer outcomes.

While 5FU was discovered in 1957 and was proven an effective treatment in metastatic colorectal cancer in 1968, it was not until the 1980s that 5FU became clearly established as the only safe and effective systemic, adjuvant, and metastatic therapy for colon cancer. When administered to patients with metastatic colon cancer it improved median survival from 6 to 11 months. When administered to patients with stage III, node-positive colon cancer it decreased the relative relapse rate by 30%. 5FU remained the only safe and effective systemic therapy until the dawn of the new millennium. In 1999, with the FDA approval of Irinotecan, the landscape of systemic colon cancer therapy changed, and boy did it change. Within a span of seven years, six new drugs, three chemotherapy and three targeted therapy, were found to be active in colon cancer. Combination chemotherapy was not just making an impact it was more than doubling the survival rate of patients with metastatic colon cancer. When used in the adjuvant setting, combination chemotherapy, which had become the standard of care in nearly all other organ cancers, was finally paying dividends in colon cancer treatment as well. The benefit of chemotherapy was not only proven in node-postive disease but also suggested in high-risk, node-negative disease. Improvements were not limited to increases in cure and survival but also included quality of life, as a new category of treatments, support drugs, was introduced. Finally, the three newly approved targeted therapies that were increasing the survival of patients with metastatic colon cancer raised the possibility of higher cure rates for adjuvant patients.

By 2005, Irinotecan, Oxaliplatin, Bevacizumab, and Cetuximab had been approved. When all of these new treatments were used, the life expectancy of patients with metastatic colon cancer was prolonged beyond 2 years. After 30 years of false starts and empty promises, in a span of just 5 years, patients with metastatic colorectal cancer witnessed a more than doubling of mean survival from 11 to 25 months. By 2005, Oxaliplatin, when added to 5FU, had also been proven to further decrease the relative relapse rate to 40% in patients with node-positive disease.

Adding complexity to the selection of an optimal treatment strategy are two other newly approved drugs: CAPECITABINE (XELODA), an oral form of 5-Fluorouracil and Panitumimab (Vectibix), an EGFR inhibitor. Prior research confirmed that the clinical benefit of 5FU could be enhanced if it was administered by continuous intravenous infusion. Unfortunately, the process of continuous infusion requires a stable long-term venous access. The most common type of long-term access is a surgically implanted venous PORT. Once the port is placed, patients receive the continuous infusion of 5FU through a small portable pump. The complexity, cost, and risks of this approach stimulated research into an orally bio-available form of 5FU so that a daily oral dosing schedule could mimic continuous intravenous infusion. Capecitabine is the result.

This newly expanded arsenal of weapons to be used in the fight against colon cancer is producing an ever-increasing volume of medical research and has resulted in some very provocative phase 2 (evaluating the effectiveness of treatment) results. Unfortunately, phase 2 clinical trial results leave many unanswered questions for the patients of this new millennium. What is the role of each agent in the management of colon cancer? How and when should each drug be incorporated? How should these new drugs be combined and/or sequenced? What role will these new targeted therapies have in the adjuvant setting? Results from phase 2 testing, regardless of the enthusiasm with which they are reported, still require phase 3 testing for conclusive proof of superiority over the current standard of care to warrant a change in that standard of care. Unfortunately, phase 3 testing of adjuvant treatments may take five to seven years to complete, leaving the physician and the patient to grapple with unproven treatment options.

I presented Eric and Kim my treatment recommendation, which happened to be a nationally conducted clinical trial. I thought that this study represented Eric's best option, as it not only offered Eric the standard-of-care chemotherapy treatment with 5FU plus Oxaliplatin, but also, it offered the possibility of him receiving an additional therapy—an additional therapy that had been proven effective in the metastatic setting.

My conversation with Doris and Sam followed a similar course, with one exception. I also had to explain that unlike the colon cancer research, which focused on systemic relapse, rectal cancer research was equally concerned with loco-regional recurrence. Once again, cooperative research groups like the NSABP paved the road to progress. In the NSABP clinical trial identified as R-01, surgery was compared to surgery plus radiation and to surgery plus 5FU-based chemotherapy. R-01 demonstrated that surgery plus 5FU-based chemotherapy could decrease systemic relapse and surgery plus radiation could decrease local recurrence. Successful clinical trials by NSABP and other cooperative research groups subsequently proved that concurrent postoperative chemotherapy plus radiation therapy was superior to either postoperative adjuvant modality alone. Subsequent trials demonstrated that patient outcomes could be further improved by giving 5FU continuously during radiation rather than by intermittent intravenous infusion. Meanwhile, cooperative research groups in Europe conducted similar clinical trials but in these trials the concurrent chemotherapy plus radiation therapy was administered before surgery. These European trials demonstrated similar improved outcomes (decreased local recurrence and decreased systemic relapse) but also increased sphincter sparing via LAR. By 2005, a consensus built that all endoscopic ultrasound-proven T2, N1 or more advanced rectal cancers undergo preoperative combined treatment with concurrent infusional 5FU plus radiation followed by LAR surgery, if feasible, then followed by additional 5FU therapy to complete a total of six months of 5FU. Research would now focus on the addition of the new systemic therapies to the 5FU plus radiation platform.

Doris and Sam took their usual optimistic outlook. The endoscopic ultrasound suggested the tumor extended through the muscularis but the nodes appeared uninvolved. They were ready to get on with treatment and not inclined to pursue a clinical trial. Eric and Kim, on the other hand, who are half Doris and Sam's age weren't willing to leave any stone unturned. They were inclined to participate in a clinical trial. But before Eric could be enrolled, he would need to sign an informed consent document that attests to his complete understanding of all potential risks and benefits associated with the treatment outlined in the clinical trial. This was the beginning of the second most difficult job I have as a medical oncologist, explaining and comparing the risks and benefits of a clinical trial with standard treatment.

The Language Of Clinical Outcomes

Explaining treatment risks and benefits can be complicated in the best of situations. Unfortunately, because medical researchers have not standardized the language of treatment-related measures and outcomes, this process can be a nightmare. The language of the oncologist can be very confusing. Even the word "cancer" is not uniformly used but may be substituted by malignant growth, cancerous tumor, NEOPLASM, etc. The outcomes of treatment are even more confusing for patients to understand as terms such as REMISSION, RESPONSE, RECURRENCE, PROGRESSION, and SURVIVAL are used to express the outcomes of therapy. Worse, for each of these outcomes like remission or response, a myriad of qualifiers will be added, including minor, partial, complete, clinical, radiographic, and pathologic. The terms progression and survival may be used in conjunction with or as an alternative to remission and response and then further refined or more likely confused by qualifying descriptions such as FREEDOM FROM PROGRESSION, RELAPSE-FREE PROGRESSION, TIME TO PROGRESSION, OVERALL SURVIVAL, and DISEASE-SPECIFIC SURVIVAL. If this was not confusing enough, these outcome measurements are reported as statistical probabilities, which are usually relative rather than absolute. It often sounds like double talk. How can patients and their loved ones be expected to understand? They just want to know if they will be cured.

Unbelievably, it gets worse. Many different clinical trials are conducted on each specific treatment to evaluate its effectiveness and to generate outcomes, but because the trial designs are not identical, the results are not either. The oncologist not only has to present this confusing data with confusing words but also he or she may have to present it for two or three trials, none of which used the same outcomes or reached the same conclusions.

In this era of patient empowerment and shared decision making, after the dizzying display of data, the doctor is supposed to ask the patient what he or she wants to do. The thoroughly confused patient often responds, "What would you recommend to your wife or mother?"

It does not have to be this way, and it should not. It is clear to me after 20 years of caring for cancer patients that there needs to be a consensus among oncologists on how data are reported and presented so that they are meaningful, the discussed risks and benefits are absolute, and the data can be compared. Fortunately for patients with breast and colon cancer, a research group led by Dr. Peter Ravdin, has published such an approach. It has been made available to patients and physicians through an Internet site: *www.adjuvantonline.com.* I have begun using this simple method, which poses the question: "What would happen to 100 patients such as yourself if…" The approach is straightforward and can be quite illuminating, as my discussion with Eric and Kim illustrates. The questions Eric, Kim, and I posed were as follows: What would happen to 100 people like Eric if after his surgery he did no further treatment? What would happen to 100 people like Eric if he received a 5FU adjuvant treatment only? What would happen to 100 people like Eric if he received combination chemo-therapy with Oxaliplatin in addition to 5FU?

Answers to these questions are made possible by a computer analysis, which creates an age- and risk factor-adjusted assessment of cancer cure based on a huge dataset, including all relevant phase 3 clinical trials. This type of data compari-son where many related but not identical clinical trials are combined is called a META-ANALYSIS and is very valuable in assessing risk in a cancer population.

Eric and Kim were very computer literate and loved the concept. A com-puter-generated mathematical model seemed to provide a certain comfort and validation, as if they were being provided an expert second opinion. I find many patients respond this way. Unfortunately such modeling is currently only avail-able to patients with breast and colon cancers. Cancers of the prostate, lung, ovary, etc., and rectal cancers like Doris's lack a similar database for analysis. For those patients, like Doris and Sam, I have to summarize the evidence as best I can. But for patients with breast or colon cancer like Eric, the analysis begins by sitting together at the computer and entering the necessary data. The online program requests information about the patient and final pathology. We huddled close as I typed in Eric's age and TNM staging. All that was left to do was to hit "enter," and then the computer analysis would be underway.

The first question posed was this: Over the next five years, what would happen to 100 people like Eric if they chose no adjuvant systemic treatment? Studies suggest 76 would be cured by the surgery, free of cancer. Twenty-three of the remaining 24 individuals with colon cancer would relapse and die.

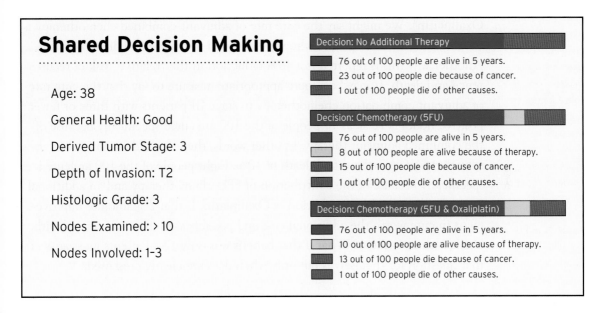

Shared Decision Making

Age: 38

General Health: Good

Derived Tumor Stage: 3

Depth of Invasion: T2

Histologic Grade: 3

Nodes Examined: > 10

Nodes Involved: 1-3

Decision: No Additional Therapy
- 76 out of 100 people are alive in 5 years.
- 23 out of 100 people die because of cancer.
- 1 out of 100 people die of other causes.

Decision: Chemotherapy (5FU)
- 76 out of 100 people are alive in 5 years.
- 8 out of 100 people are alive because of therapy.
- 15 out of 100 people die because of cancer.
- 1 out of 100 people die of other causes.

Decision: Chemotherapy (5FU & Oxaliplatin)
- 76 out of 100 people are alive in 5 years.
- 10 out of 100 people are alive because of therapy.
- 13 out of 100 people die because of cancer.
- 1 out of 100 people die of other causes.

Figure 4-6: Adjuvantonline: Shared Decision Making

One person would likely die of a cause unrelated to the colon cancer. Most unfortunately, the majority of those who relapse would eventually die from the colon cancer.

The second question posed in the computer analysis was this: Over the next five years, what would happen to 100 people like Eric if they chose adjuvant 5FU therapy? Studies suggest that eight fewer people would relapse. Eighty-four people would be alive, well, and free of cancer; however, 15 would have relapsed, likely to die of cancer.

The third question posed in the computer survey was this: What would happen to 100 people like Eric if adjuvant combination chemotherapy with a 5FU plus Oxaliplatin regimen were used? Studies suggest that the chemotherapy would save the lives of 10 people. Eighty-six people would be alive and well, free of cancer relapse, whereas 13 people would succumb to the cancer (Figure 4-6).

An oncologist might review this information on surgery followed by chemotherapy and report that the overall cure rate is 86%, but that would not explain the specific contribution of each component of therapy (surgery, 5FU,

Oxaliplatin). We might say the cure rate of adjuvant-combined chemotherapy is 40% because 10 of 23 people who were destined to relapse and die were cured. Another way this is reported is a 40% reduction in the "relative" risk of recurrence and death. It may be a more appropriate measure to say that the cure rate of adjuvant combination chemotherapy in stage III patients with three or fewer positive nodes is 10%, as 10 people of the 100 are cured specifically because of the combined adjuvant therapy. In other words, there is a reduction in the "absolute" risk of recurrence and death of 10%. Eight people of the 100 are cured specifically because of the contribution of 5FU chemotherapy and an additional 2 people are cured by the addition of Oxaliplatin. Is that 2% absolute improvement in cure worth the additional cost and possible side effects associated with Oxaliplatin treatment? What if that benefit was only 1%? Patients must answer that question for themselves but only when data are clearly presented.

When the data are presented in this way, it becomes clear that only 10 people receiving adjuvant therapy will truly benefit from the treatment, yet all 100 will be treated. As I explained to Eric and Kim, science has yet to develop technology that can detect micrometastases. There is no way to know who are the 76 people already cured by the surgery or who are the 13 people destined to relapse despite taking chemotherapy. Thus, all 100 people are treated: 76 who have no need because they are cured by surgery, 13 who have no need because adjuvant chemotherapy will not help them, and 10 who will be truly cured by this intervention.

Eric and Kim found the discussion encouraging. Undergoing outpatient chemotherapy for six months seemed a small cost to reduce, by nearly half, Eric's risk of relapse. Kim became excited when she had a sudden realization that the analysis did not include the additional therapy being studied in the clinical trial that I had recommended. Could this additional therapy further increase Eric's chance of cure? Certainly, the additional therapy is under investigation because researchers hope it will improve outcomes, but the reason that the additional therapy was not included in the analysis is that phase 3 studies evaluating its role in the adjuvant setting have not been concluded. This means that we do not currently know whether this additional therapy may benefit patients like Eric, and more importantly, we do not know what toxicities or harm this additional therapy may cause.

It seemed like a good time to review what we had just discussed. The systemic therapy of cancer has evolved by demonstrating a treatment's ability to reduce the size of the cancer and prolong life in patients with metastatic cancer, and to eradicate micrometastases and increase the number of patients cured who are treated adjuvantly. Sequential improvements in therapy have been accomplished using a standardized three-phase approach, which confirms safety (phase 1), efficacy (phase 2), and superiority (phase 3). The process of improvement is continuous such that at any moment tens of research studies are ongoing in each phase. Clinical trials not only evaluate new systemic therapies, alone and in combination, but also evaluate how to best integrate these therapies with the loco-regional modalities of surgery and radiation.

This dynamic and constantly improving treatment landscape may be exciting for researchers and may provide encouragement for those at risk like Eric, but it can also pose a dilemma for the patient and doctor who want to use all of the resources available to maximize the opportunity for cure and survival. Patients such as Eric and Doris, their loved ones, as well as their doctors often need some direction, some authority, to pronounce a current standard of care, define reasonable alternatives when a standard does not exist, and provide guidance for patients who wish to pursue a clinical trial option. This was my next topic of discussion.

The Standard Of Care

Nationally and internationally, oncologists and cancer researchers have recognized the problems that the abundance of emerging data creates for patients making treatment decisions. The oncology community has responded by creating a system for peer review, discussion, and dissemination of new research. Data are released at designated meetings and in professional peer-reviewed journals.

The oncology community has also responded by developing cooperative clinical research groups, such as the National Surgical Adjuvant Breast and Bowel Project, to provide broad patient access to new therapies in phase 2 and phase 3 testing. Consensus conferences, developed by the National Comprehensive Cancer Center Network, the American Society of Clinical Oncology, and the National Cancer Institute, have been organized to review emerging data and to provide a consensus on patient management. The following discussions reflect those most recent consensus statements on stage-specific therapies of cancers of the rectum and colon.

STAGE I RECTAL CANCER–(old stage: Dukes' A or Modified Astler-Coller A and B1): Because of its localized nature, stage I has a high cure rate. Standard treatment options are as follows:

1) Wide surgical RESECTION and ANASTOMOSIS when an adequate low anterior resection (LAR) can be performed.

2) Wide surgical resection with abdomino-perineal resection (APR) for lesions too distal to permit low anterior resection (LAR).

3) One prospective multicenter phase 2 study and several larger retrospective series suggest that local excision may be adequate for some well-staged patients with small (<4 centimeters) tumors with good histologic prognostic features: well to moderately differentiated adenocarcinomas; without lymphatic, venous, or perineural invasion. These patients may have outcomes equivalent to APR or LAR.

STAGE II RECTAL CANCER–(old stage: Dukes' B or Modified Astler-Coller B2 and B3): Standard treatment options are as follows:

1) Wide surgical resection with anal sphincter preservation via a low anterior resection (LAR) with colorectal or coloanal REANASTOMOSIS when feasible, followed by chemotherapy and postoperative radiation therapy.

2) Wide surgical resection with abdomino-perineal resection with adjuvant chemotherapy and postoperative radiation therapy.

3) Preoperative radiation therapy with or without 5FU-based chemotherapy followed by surgery with an attempt to preserve sphincter function and subsequent adjuvant chemotherapy to complete six months of adjuvant 5FU.

STAGE III RECTAL CANCER–(old stage: Dukes' C or Modified Astler-Coller C1 – C3): Stage III rectal cancer denotes disease with lymph node involvement. The number of positive lymph nodes affects PROGNOSIS. Patients with one to three involved nodes have superior survival to those with four or more involved nodes. Standard treatment options are as follows:

1) Wide surgical resection with low anterior resection (LAR) with colorectal or coloanal reanastomosis when feasible, followed by chemotherapy and postoperative radiation therapy.

2) Wide surgical resection with abdomino-perineal resection with adjuvant chemotherapy and postoperative radiation therapy.

3) Preoperative radiation therapy with or without 5FU-based chemotherapy followed by surgery with an attempt to preserve sphincter function with subsequent adjuvant chemotherapy.

4) Clinical trials evaluating new drugs and biological therapy.

STAGE IV RECTAL CANCER–(old stage: Modified Astler-Coller D): Standard treatment options are as follows:

1) Surgical resection/anastomosis or bypass of obstructing lesions in selected cases or resection for PALLIATION.

2) Surgical resection of isolated metastases.

3) Chemoradiation for local palliation.

4) Chemotherapy alone for distant disease after resection of local disease.

5) Clinical trials evaluating new drugs and biological therapy.

RECURRENT RECTAL CANCER–Standard treatment options are as follows:

1) Resection of locally recurrent rectal cancer may be palliative or curative in selected patients.

2) Resection of liver metastases in selected patients (the five-year cure rate with resection of solitary metastases exceeds 20%).

3) Resection of isolated pulmonary or ovarian metastases.

4) Palliative radiation therapy.

5) Palliative chemotherapy.

STAGE 0 COLON CANCER–Carcinoma in situ: Treatment options are as follows:

1) Local excision or simple polypectomy with clear margins.

2) Colon resection for larger lesions not amenable to local excision.

STAGE I COLON CANCER–(old stage: Dukes' A or Modified Astler-Collier A and B): Because of its localized nature, stage I has a high cure rate. Treatment options are as follows:

1) Wide surgical resection and anastomosis. The role of laparoscopic techniques in the treatment of colon cancer is under evaluation in a multicenter prospective randomized trial comparing laparoscopic-assisted colectomy (LAC) with open colectomy.[3]

STAGE II COLON CANCER–(old stage: Dukes' B or Modified Astler-Collier B2 and B3): Treatment options are as follows:

1) Wide surgical resection and anastomosis. The role of laparoscopic techniques in the treatment of colon cancer remains under evaluation.

[3] Laprascopic-assisted colectomy has many proponents and practitioners, but it remains investigational as results from phase 3 trials have not been published.

2) Following surgery, patients should be considered for entry into carefully controlled clinical trials evaluating the use of systemic or regional chemotherapy, radiation therapy, or biologic therapy.

Adjuvant Therapy:

Research shows that some subgroups of patients with stage II colon cancer may be at higher-than-average risk for recurrence (including those with anatomic features such as tumor adherence to adjacent structures, perforation, or complete obstruction, or with biologic characteristics such as aneuploidy, elevated CEA, and high S-phase). Adjuvant 5FU-based chemotherapy improves overall survival in these patients. However, investigators from the National Surgical Adjuvant Breast and Bowel Project have indicated that the reduction in risk of recurrence by adjuvant therapy in patients with stage II disease is of similar magnitude to the benefit seen in patients with treated stage III disease. Therefore, though an overall survival advantage has not been established for all stage II patients, they suggest *all* stage II patients undergo adjuvant therapy.

STAGE III COLON CANCER–(old stage: Dukes' C or Modified Astler-Collier C1 – C3): Stage III colon cancer denotes lymph node involvement. Studies have indicated that the number of lymph nodes involved affects prognosis. Patients with one to three involved nodes have superior survival to those with four or more involved nodes. Treatment options are as follows:

1) Wide surgical resection and anastomosis. The role of laparoscopic techniques in the treatment of colon cancer is under evaluation in a multicenter prospective randomized trial comparing laparoscopic-assisted colectomy (LAC) with open colectomy. Patients who are not candidates for clinical trials should receive postoperative chemotherapy with Fluorouracil (5FU)-Leucovorin for six months. Based on results from the M.O.S.A.I.C. trial presented at the American Society of Clinical Oncology meeting in 2003, adjuvant 5FU plus Oxaliplatin adjuvant chemotherapy regimens became the new standard.

2) Eligible patients should be considered for entry into carefully controlled clinical trials comparing various postoperative chemotherapy

regimens. These trials also now include Oxaliplatin-based and Irino-tecan-based chemotherapy with new-targeted agents.

STAGE IV AND RECURRENT COLON CANCER–(old stage: Dukes' Modified Astler-Collier D): Stage IV colon cancer denotes distant metastatic disease. Treatment of recurrent colon cancer depends on the sites of recurrent disease demonstrable by physical examination and/or radiographic studies. Treatment options are as follows:

1) Surgical resection of locally recurrent cancer.

2) Surgical resection/anastomosis or bypass of obstructing or bleeding primary lesions in selected metastatic cases.

3) Resection of liver metastases in selected metastatic patients. (The five-year cure rate with resection of solitary or combination metastases exceeds 20%.) ABLATION in selected patients.

4) Resection of isolated pulmonary, ovarian, or liver metastases in selected patients.

5) Palliative radiation therapy.

6) Palliative systemic therapy (chemotherapy and targeted therapy).

7) Clinical trials evaluating new drugs and biological/targeted therapy.

8) Clinical trials comparing various chemotherapy regimens or biological/targeted therapy, alone or in a combination.

Metastatic Therapy:

Locally recurrent colon cancer, such as a SUTURE LINE or ANASTOMOSIS SITE recurrence, may be resectable. Approximately 40% of colon cancer patients will be diagnosed with HEPATIC METASTASES either at the time of initial presentation or as a result of disease recurrence. However, only a small proportion of patients with hepatic metastases are candidates for surgical resection. Advances in tumor ablation techniques and in systemic therapy provide a number of treatment options.

For patients with hepatic metastasis considered to be resectable (based on the number of lesions, locations of lesions, lack of major vascular involvement, absent or limited EXTRAHEPATIC disease, and sufficient FUNCTIONAL HEPATIC RESERVE), a negative margin resection has resulted in five-year survival rates of 25% to 40% in mostly nonrandomized studies.

For patients with hepatic metastases deemed unresectable, RADIO FREQUENCY ABLATION has emerged as a safe technique (2% major morbidity and <1% mortality rate) that may provide long-term tumor control. Other local ablative techniques that have been used to manage liver metastases include EMBOLIZATION, CRYOSURGERY, and INTERSTITIAL RADIATION THERAPY. Patients with limited pulmonary metastases and patients with both limited pulmonary and hepatic metastases may also be considered for surgical resection, with five-year survival possible in highly selected patients.

Recommended first-line chemotherapy treatment for patients with advanced colorectal cancer include combination 5FU chemotherapy with either Oxaliplatin or Irinotecan in addition to Bevacizumab.

Second-line chemotherapy treatment for patients who progress after first-line chemotherapy is guided by which treatment was used for first-line treatment. Patients who were treated with an Oxaliplatin-containing regimen should be treated with an Irinotecan-based regimen, and patients who already received an Irinotecan-based regimen should be treated with an Oxaliplatin-based regimen. If Irinotecan is used and resistance is observed, Cetuximab or Panitumimab may be used.

The rapid expansion of the arsenal of systemic weapons to fight cancer of the colon and rectum leaves many questions regarding optimum combinations and sequencing. Clinical trials will be critical to resolve theses questions. What is clear, at least for patients with advanced disease, is that those who are exposed to all of the systemic therapies currently available enjoy the longest survival.

Shared Decision Making

After a bit more deliberation, participating in the clinical trial seemed like a reasonable solution to all of Kim's concerns, but Eric seemed hesitant. He was concerned that he might enroll in the trial but not receive the additional therapy. Eric was correct. In order to prove that a therapeutic drug adds benefit, clinical trials are structured so that some of the patients receive the current standard of care, whereas others receive the standard treatment plus the additional therapy under investigation. This kind of trial design is the most common and is referred to as RANDOMIZED, where patients are randomly assigned to receive either the standard treatment arm or the arm evaluating the risk/benefit of the additional therapy. Kim did not understand why I could not give Eric standard treatment plus the additional therapy because she knew another patient in my office who was receiving the "additional therapy drug" who was not on a clinical trial. I explained that my other patient had advanced cancer for which the additional therapy was approved but it was not approved for Eric's stage of cancer. Giving therapies to patients before they are approved is risky, as clinical trials not only evaluate the reduction in risk of recurrence but also the negative aspects of new therapies, such as side effects and complications. The only way Eric could receive the additional therapy was by participating in a clinical trial and only then if he was randomized to the investigational arm.

After one more night to sleep on their decision, Eric and Kim signed the informed consent. The following Monday, after all necessary tests were completed per the clinical trial requirements, treatment was begun. Blood tests, additional x-rays, and a test to measure Eric's heart function had been performed, and fortunately, no abnormalities were detected. Eric was randomized to receive the investigational additional therapy as well as the standard chemotherapy.

For Doris and Sam the discussion progressed along similar lines. I reiterated that the current standard of care in stage II or III rectal cancer was definitive surgery with perioperative 5FU plus radiation followed by 5FU alone to complete six months adjuvant chemotherapy. I explained that although the jury was still out, due to pending phase 3 data, the emerging evidence favored the preoperative use of continuous intravenous 5FU plus radiation, which would necessitate the placement of a port. I also explained the emerging role of Oxali-platin in the adjuvant therapy of colon cancer and the newly approved targeted therapies to treat metastatic colorectal cancer. I then reviewed the clinical trials evaluating these new agents as additional therapy for which Doris may be eligi-ble. Doris and Sam were appreciative of my time and the information I provided but their minds were made up. I recommended they relate their decision to ex-clude the clinical trial option to their children, who had been both supportive and involved in the decision process thus far. Sam said they all met last evening and were 100% behind whatever Doris decided. Doris was comfortable with her decision to proceed with preop continuous infusion 5FU and concurrent radiation therapy. This treatment plan gave her a greater than 80% probability of cure if our CT scans, exam, and ultrasound correctly diagnosed a T3 N0 M0 tumor. I referred her to INTERVENTIONAL RADIOLOGY for a port, and I called Drs. Drake and Armstrong to notify them of Doris's decision and outlined the tentative treatment schedule for all involved.

For my patients like Doris and Eric and their families, the final treatment decision generates a collective sigh of relief. Positive attitudes usually prevail over the fears and anxieties of treatment side effects once treatment begins. However, patients at this point usually have new questions. I will address the most common ones in Section III.

More Questions

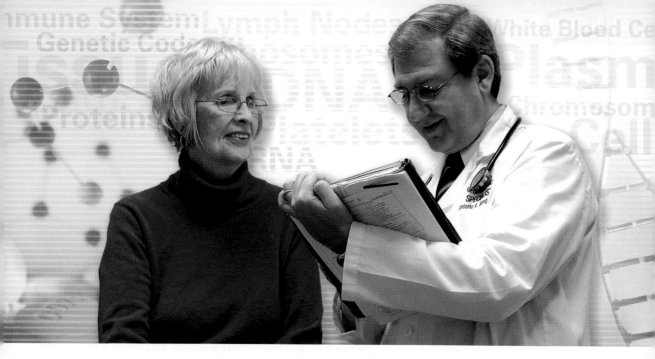

Introduction

The shock of a cancer diagnosis and the wealth of information presented to patients in the weeks and months immediately following the pronouncement "you have cancer" are numbing. Often, as patients become accustomed to the routine of adjuvant therapy, they wish to discuss many issues that the care team began to address before initiating treatment as well as new concerns about diet, exercise, sexuality, and living with a cancer diagnosis. In this section I discuss some of the more common themes my patients voice: the issues of CANCER PREVENTION, TREATMENT SURVEILLANCE, and CANCER RELAPSE. We begin with the question next asked by Kim, wouldn't Eric benefit from ALTERNATIVE THERAPIES?

Chapter Five

Alternative Therapies

Shortly after initiating Eric's treatment, Kim called regarding an article in the newspaper that praised a new wonder drug for colon cancer. The "wonder drug" discussion raised the broader question of how a patient and their supportive family members remain sane amidst the endless reports of break-throughs, miracles, and cures. There is no easy answer. In my observation, the key to sanity can be found in a patient's trust in the integrity of his or her care-giver and faith in his or her own judgment. All patients will reach a line in the sand when they have to decide on treatment. Only by believing that they have performed adequate due diligence and by trusting their caregivers' recommenda-tions can that decision be made without regret. Eric and Kim went through such a process. I believed they had a foundation of faith and trust that would keep them sane in the coming months and years.

Kim also raised the possibility of pursuing alternative therapy. Thankfully, before embarking on such an initiative, they consulted with me. I thought some definitions were needed to help us structure the discussion. Unconventional, alternative, or COMPLEMENTARY THERAPIES encompass a broad spectrum of practices and beliefs and are, therefore, very difficult to define. What is com-mon to these therapies is that they do not conform with the beliefs or standards of the conventional mainstream medical establishment or accepted standard of care. These standards can also be culturally dependent, which may create further confusion, i.e., traditional Chinese medicine is considered unconventional in the United States, whereas it is a standard practice in China. Also, with uncon-ventional therapies, their proof of effectiveness is most often conveyed through personal anecdote rather than stringent evidence-based criteria reached through multiphase clinical research.

Unconventional therapies may be subdivided into COMPLEMENTARY THERAPIES and ALTERNATIVE THERAPIES. Complementary therapies can be further categorized as spiritual, psychological, nutritional, and physical. Meditation, relaxation, imaging, prayer, massage, and dietary supplements would be just a few of the interventions included in this vital quartet of complementary therapies. These approaches to healing are not in conflict with conventional Western medicine; rather, in most cases, they can be effectively integrated into standard medical practice. Alternative therapies, as the name implies, are not intended to be integrated into conventional therapy; rather, they are offered as a complete therapy. Unproven by evidence-based criteria, pharmacologic treatments comprise the bulk of alternative therapies. These therapies are particularly susceptible to quackery, and false and excessive claims and high-profit motives are common.

The increased interest in and attractiveness of unconventional therapies are understandable. The technologic and frequently impersonal nature of modern medicine leaves patients feeling lost and empty. Insensitive, hurried interactions with physicians often result in patients feeling helpless, out of control, and ignored. The confusing jargon and statistics further alienate the patient and family. Finally, the cold, hard truth of some cancer diagnoses and the limited effectiveness of some conventional standard therapies may foster hopelessness. Unconventional medicine, on the other hand, is perceived as natural, simpler, nontoxic, and more understandable. Its practitioners are viewed as more caring and their approach more holistic. The absence of data eliminates the difficult discussions of toxicity, response, and survival probability.

Eric asked, "How does one evaluate and choose an unconventional approach to healing?" There are a few guidelines that I suggest my patients follow. First, avoid any practitioner of any unconventional (or for that matter mainstream) method who is evasive. People who are practicing healing techniques that they believe in will want to share them with your other doctors, not hide them. Second, avoid treatments that are touted to work only if you stop your traditional treatments. Especially with cancer treatment, we need to take advantage of all treatments that may help. Third, avoid practitioners who have exclusive access to the cure but will not tell anyone what it is. Practitioners who truly believe in what they are doing want to share their successes. Fourth, beware of the motivations of the people making recommendations.

It is unusual for natural healing techniques to be very expensive. If an exclusive treatment is being suggested and is very expensive, examine the motivations of the prescriber. Be aware that most unconventional therapies are not covered by insurance, given the absence of supporting data from well-designed clinical trials. Finally, pick an unconventional therapy that you feel good enough about to discuss with your physician. Your participation in restoring or maintaining your health is absolutely essential. The success of many alternative treatments depends in great part on your belief in the potential of the therapy to improve your health. If you truly believe in the therapy, be willing to discuss it not only with your family and friends, but also with your physician.

Eric and Kim seemed comfortable with my response. I told them that if they came across a particularly appealing complementary treatment to bring it to my attention for discussion. As I was about to leave the room, I noticed Eric appeared uneasy. I asked again if he was comfortable with his treatment decision. He said that this was not what was troubling him. He said he worried about his sister's risk of colon cancer even though his cancer was so unlikely to be hereditary. I told him that there were steps his sister could take right now to reduce her risk of getting cancer.

Chapter 6

Prevention

S trategies are being designed that may help to prevent first and subsequent colorectal cancers. These strategies include lifestyle modifications, genetic testing, preventative medication, and most importantly screening. Diet and exercise may also play an important role in prevention. Dietary fats, especially from grilled meats, as well as inadequate fiber, calcium, and selenium intake are all being investigated as possible factors that increase the risk of colon cancer. Studies of both men and women have suggested that three or more hours of vigorous exercise a week may significantly reduce the risk of developing cancer in general. The implication of a dietary factor/sedentary behavior relationship to cancer is based on population studies. For example, countries with very low breast cancer incidence, like Japan, also have very low-fat diets, but when Japanese people emigrate to the U.S. and assume a Western diet, within two generations their offspring's breast cancer incidence matches the general U.S. population. The common adult cancers of Western countries are less frequently observed in the developing world where diets are more vegetable based and people are much less sedentary. Unfortunately, such population studies are at best suggestive. Proof of relationships between diet, exercise, and cancer requires research that both confirms and explains the relationship.

A great deal of research has also been focused on developing drugs that can prevent cancer. The preventative treatment of cancer with a drug is called CHEMOPREVENTION. One drug, called Tamoxifen (Nolvadex), which interferes with natural estrogen, has now been approved for the chemoprevention of breast cancer. Early research suggests that in high-risk women, breast cancers may be reduced by as much as 50% with medications, like Tamoxifen, that interfere with estrogen. Unfortunately, no similar drug has yet been proven effective in colorectal cancer prevention, but aspirin-like compounds, technically called Cox-1 and Cox-2 inhibitor drugs, have demonstrated some very exciting results in preliminary testing. Unfortunately, every medication also poses risks; the potential cardiac risk of Cox-2 inhibitors has clouded the water regarding their role in prevention. Even after a medication has been proven to have preventative properties and is deemed both safe and effective, who should receive chemoprevention and for how long remains to be established.

Clearly the best prevention strategy is following screening guidelines. Unfortunately, for reasons discussed earlier, those guidelines are followed by less than half the population. Thus despite clear guidelines, healthcare experts are confronted by patients who demand the potentially risky and still-unproven pill over the recommended screening colonoscopy.

Making fateful decisions that depend on medical science as well as highly personal judgments about how future illness will affect quality of life is difficult at best. Neither doctor nor patient can do it alone. With colon cancer chemoprevention, clinicians and patients need to understand the limits of what we know and what we can control about the future. Patients and their doctors who work at making good decisions together will be far more likely to make the best use of what current medical science has to offer.

Chapter 7

Advanced and Relapsed Cancer

Eric and Kim had raised the "what if" question about relapse. I had hoped to avoid this discussion, as it can be unpleasant to talk about treatment failure, which was unlikely given Eric's probability of cure. Occasionally, cancer will recur only in the ANASTOMOTIC SITE within the colon. In these cases, it is referred to as a LOCAL RECURRENCE and is likely curable. However, most relapses are systemic, which means they are metastases. Metastases are rarely cured. I could not think of a gentle way to approach metastatic cancer and thus I decided to detour for a bit, beginning the discussion with locally and regionally recurrent cancer, a subject that I neglected in our earlier discussion.

Locally Recurrent Cancer

I have previously focused on people who undergo surgical removal of the colorectal tumor and subsequent adjuvant therapy to destroy micrometastases and reduce the risk of relapse. These people are said to have localized cancer, and consensus guidelines offer reasonable clarity in the approach to management. I'll now discuss the patient with locally or regionally recurrent colorectal cancer. Reports suggest that despite the available treatment options, up to 25% of stage II and III rectal cancer patients and 5–10% of stage II and III colon cancer patients will recur loco-regionally without evidence of systemic relapse. Guidelines to direct the management of these patients are less clear; therefore, I will share where current research is leading us.

Following the completion of definitive loco-regional therapy and systemic adjuvant treatment, patients with stage II and stage III colorectal cancers remain under surveillance with serial clinical and laboratory monitoring. The surveillance is designed to detect signs or symptoms of a loco-regional recurrence or systemic relapse. The most common asymptomatic sign of a loco-regional recurrence is a rise in CEA, a nonspecific chemical marker present in the blood of approximately two-thirds of patients with colorectal cancer. The most common symptoms of a loco-regional recurrence are those related to bowel obstruction. Obstructive symptoms may be due to tumor recurrence at the site of bowel anastomosis or due to extrinsic pressure from regional lymph node metastases. A clinically suspected local recurrence or regional node relapse will require colonoscopy, CT imaging, and sometimes PET scanning to anatomically identify and distinguish an isolated loco-regional recurrence from a systemic relapse.

Suspected recurrences are usually confirmed pathologically via colonoscope biopsy, laprascope biopsy, or CT-directed needle biopsy. If the imaging studies only reveal a loco-regional recurrence, surgery is indicated. If a systemic relapse is suggested but confined to three or fewer deposits within an organ (referred to as OLIGOMETASTASES) they also may be treated for cure.

In these unique situations where a tumor has re-emerged as an isolated anastomotic recurrence, an isolated nodal recurrence, or a limited organ relapse (oligometastases) cure may still be possible using a combination of surgical resection and systemic therapy. New surgical techniques to ablate tumors are under investigation but remain experimental, as phase 3 investigation clinical trials have not been completed.

Metastatic Colon Cancer

The evaluation of patients with metastatic disease either at initial presentation or after relapse can be performed in a similar way. Unfortunately, cure is rare in metastatic disease; therefore, the most important treatment outcomes to measure are length of life and quality of life. I recommend using the percentage of people alive at one, two, three, and five years after treatment as a meaningful measure of treatment effectiveness. Survival may be the ultimate goal of treatment, but the care of the patient with metastatic disease is complicated by the need to manage disease-related symptoms. Before survival can be considered, suffering must be addressed. The ability of a treatment to reduce symptoms is measured as its response rate.

Response may be more important than survival in a suffering patient. Outcomes, such as one-year survival and clinical response are most commonly presented in relative terms but can also be presented as absolute impact in the 100-patient method described previously.

Despite all of the described methods to screen, diagnose, and adjuvantly treat colorectal cancer when it is localized, 35% of all colorectal cancer patients still die from their disease because the cancer metastasizes to the vital organs: lung, liver, and brain. They also may suffer from cancer involvement of bone, lymph nodes, and skin, as well as recurrences in the abdominal and pelvic cavity. Colorectal cancer in this setting is rarely curable, but a great deal can be done to diminish symptoms, improve quality of life, and prolong life. Therapy intended not to cure but to improve the quality of life is called PALLIATIVE.

Because all treatments have side effects, PALLIATIVE THERAPY demands a uniquely candid discussion of goals and objectives between the oncologist and patient. Expressions such as "watch and wait," "the treatment may be worse than the disease," and "win the battle but lose the war" are attempts by oncologists to metaphorically explain to the patient that when it comes to palliative therapy, more is not always better. The main objective in palliative therapy is maximal preservation of quality of life, not necessarily maximal tumor shrinkage, unless shrinkage (response) has been proven to impact directly on the quality of life or survival. It is also important not to diminish the dramatic success attained in the past decade as the survival of patients with metastatic colorectal cancer has more than doubled thanks to an unprecedented expansion of our arsenal of weapons. If these weapons are found to be equally effective in the adjuvant setting they may reduce the incidence of systemic relapse in the near future by as much as 50%.

Chapter Eight

Post-Treatment Surveillance

Consensus panels continue to recommend post-treatment follow-up for all patients with stages I, II, and III colorectal cancer. Follow-up should include performance of routine history and physical examinations, periodic CEA level checks, and colonoscopy. Surveillance with a narrative review of symptoms, physical exam, and laboratory assessment initially may be as frequent as every three months in the first few years after diagnosis. Surveillance should gradually diminish to annually beyond five years from diagnosis. However, surveillance is recommended for the life of the patient as second colon cancers as well as late relapse of past colon cancer and late adverse effects of prior treatments have been reported.

Historically, routine surveillance by BONE SCAN, CT scan and MRI scan had not been recommended, as none of these routine imaging procedures had been proven effective. Similar to the screening tests that were discussed earlier, for a surveillance method to be effective, it must be proven to be both sensitive and specific. Insensitive tests will miss abnormalities. Sensitive tests that are not specific will reveal abnormalities that are not related to the cancer, often leading to more tests, procedures, and anxiety that may not only be not helpful but seriously harmful. However, as a result of improved CT technology, surveillance guidelines for colon and rectal cancer were revised in 2005 to include annual CT scanning of the abdomen and pelvis in years one through three after diagnosis. Annual chest CT was also recommended in patients with rectal cancer.

Researchers continue to evaluate new technologies that might enhance the ability to both diagnose and predict relapse. PET scanning and other new imaging techniques as well as genetic tests are still considered investigational as routine screening tools. Genomics and proteinomics as well as microarray testing hold the greatest promise but are also investigational. These surveillance recommendations are outlined in Table 1.

Surveillance	Recommendations
History and Physical with Risk Assessment	Coordinating physician visits should occur every 3-6 months for the first 3 years, every 6 months during years 3 and 5, and subsequently at the discretion of the physician. Physician visits should focus on the initial risk assessment followed by the implementation of a surveillance strategy and periodic counseling based on estimated risk and feasibility of surgical interventions.
Blood Tests	
Carcinoembryonic Antigen (CEA)	Postoperative serum CEA testing should be performed every 3 months for at least 3 years after diagnosis, if the patient is a candidate for surgery or systemic therapy. (Adjuvant treatment should be completed before surveillance is initiated, as Fluorouracil-based therapy may falsely elevate CEA levels.)
Routine Blood Tests	Routine complete blood counts. Liver function tests are not routinely recommended.
Fecal Occult Blood Test	Periodic fecal occult blood testing is not recommended.
Imaging Studies	
Computerized Tomography (CT)	CT of the abdomen and chest should be done annually for 3 years for patients who are at high risk of recurrence and who could be candidates for curative-intent surgery. CT of the pelvis should be considered for patients with rectal cancer.
Chest X-Ray	Yearly chest x-rays are not recommended.
Endoscopic Procedures	
Colonoscopy	Colonoscopy should be done for all patients with colon and rectal cancer for the preoperative or postoperative documentation of a cancer-free and polyp-free colon. Following the surgical treatment for colorectal cancer, colonoscopy should be done at 3 years and if the findings are normal, every 5 years thereafter. For patients with high-risk genetic syndromes, the American Gastroenterological Association guidelines should be followed.
Flexible Proctosigmoidoscopy (Rectal Cancer)	Flexible sigmoidoscopy every 6 months for 5 years for patients who were not treated with radiation to the pelvis and who are not undergoing surveillance by colonoscopy.
Laboratory-Derived Prognostic and Predictive Factors	Until prospective data are available, use of molecular or cellular markers should not influence the surveillance strategy.

Table 1. Summary of Recommendations in "Colorectal Cancer Surveillance-2005 Update of an American Society of Clinical Oncology Practice Guideline"

Epilogue

During the next few months, Eric and Kim slowly settled into the reality of therapy. The first six weeks were the toughest, as they dealt with the rigors of treatment, the office visits, the questions and advice from family and friends, and the side effects of chemotherapy. The emotional impact of treatment overwhelmed Eric more than the physical effects. It's not easy to confront mortality at any age, and in Eric's case, certainly not at age 38. Kim and Eric's parents' doting and well-intentioned support only worsened Eric's sense of vulnerability. He became clinically depressed. I recommended counseling and an antidepressant. He agreed.

The observations from Doris and Sam were not very different. The port placement was uncomplicated and the portable infusion pump took a bit of getting used to but became second nature. Eight weeks into preoperative concurrent 5FU plus radiation Doris's bottom was sore, it burned when she passed water, and her stools were frequent and watery, but there had been no blood for weeks. Surgery was scheduled eight weeks after the conclusion of radiation treatments.

Doris underwent successful LAR surgery as planned. Pathologic review of the rectum defined Doris's tumor as T2 N0 M0, suggesting the chemo-radiation reduced the cancer from the T3 depth defined by ultrasound. Unfortunately, Dr. Armstrong felt a temporary colostomy was needed to prevent contamination of the colo-anal anastomosis, and Doris accepted that in stride as she had everything else. She returned to my clinic four weeks after surgery, still trying to adapt to the colostomy appliance, to complete her 5FU treatment. Once 5FU was completed Dr. Armstrong would reverse her colostomy.

Three months into systemic therapy, Eric seemed to turn a corner. Counseling and antidepressant therapy were helping. His treatment tolerance improved and the surgery-related pain resolved. He was mostly bothered by a sense of fatigue that he likened to that experienced during his recovery from the flu two years ago. He was beginning to feel that the worst was behind him and that life might return to normal.

Near the conclusion of chemotherapy, Eric experienced an emotional setback. I thought he would approach the day of his last treatment with elation, but surprisingly, once again he seemed depressed. Our conversation uncovered a growing emotional dependency on his active treatment as his protection against a cancer relapse. I explained that his chemotherapy had accomplished what was intended and that it was time to proceed with surveillance.

One year from that fateful day when the words "you have cancer" forever changed the lives of Eric and Doris, they were happy and healthy once again. Selective memory and the healing effects of time proved to be an effective salve to the physical and emotional wounds inflicted by the cancer diagnosis. Like millions of Americans, Eric and Doris found that they had what it takes to be cancer survivors.

My only remaining question as I close this discussion of colon cancer answers is on the lighter side: Did I have what it takes to survive a classroom of 15 second-graders? As you recall, I left Daniel's room contemplating what kind of cancer machine to demonstrate and what memento I could leave for the class. I decided Legos were a more than adequate prop for my presentation. After all, a 2-ton linear accelerator would not fit through the classroom door.

What to give second-graders was a bigger challenge. I contacted Ken, a pharmaceutical representative, who said he could donate some promotional fanny-packs. His company's marketing department developed the fanny-pack filled with exercise-related items including a water bottle, towel, and dollar-store stopwatch to create the notion that his company's fatigue-busting drug for cancer patients could get them back into exercising. I was elated as I realized that a fanny-pack bulging with all this junk would be the best give-away that any parent could bring.

The day arrived, and before curious eyes, Daniel and I entered the classroom with Legos and fanny-packs. Daniel's teacher brought the class to order, then asked Daniel to introduce me.

Daniel's introduction was the essence of brevity. "This is my dad."

The kids were great. They were attentive, well behaved and—believe it or not—interested. Upon the conclusion of my demonstration, the teacher asked the students if they had any questions. The hands shot up. I was overwhelmed at the response and pointed to a boy in the back row. He asked, "What's the best thing about your job?" I said, "It's nice to be able to help people." More hands soared. "What's the worst part of your job?" I explained that I'm not able to make all the sick people who see me feel better. More hands went up, and my head was swelling to the size of a watermelon. "What's the best part of your job?" I said, "In addition to helping people I get to come home at night and play with Daniel." I looked at Daniel; he was beaming. More hands. "What's the worst part of your job?" I may be gullible, but I'm not stupid. "Is there anyone with a question other than what is the best or worst part of my job?" I was praying that just one hand would still be up, but none were. They were all shills, asking the questions planted by their teacher.

Once again, children humbled me. I thanked the teacher and said good-bye to the class. As I left, I looked over my shoulder to see Daniel grinning ear to ear.

Glossary

5-Fluorouracil: a pyrimidine analog, $C_4H_3FN_2O_2$, used in the treatment of certain cancers.

Abdomen: the part of the body that contains the stomach, small intestine, colon, rectum, liver, spleen, pancreas, kidneys, appendix, gallbladder, and bladder.

Abdominal: having to do with the abdomen.

Abdominal cavity: the cavity of this part of the trunk lined by the peritoneum, enclosed by the body walls, the diaphragm, and the pelvic floor, and containing the visceral organs (as the stomach, intestines, and liver).

Abdomino-perineal resection: the surgical procedure that removes the entire rectum, attaching the remaining colon to the abdominal wall forming a colostomy.

Abnormal: not normal; an abnormal lesion or growth may be cancerous, premalignant (likely to become cancer), or benign.

Acquired mutations: genetic alterations resulting from chronic physical, chemical, radiation, and natural injury to DNA; responsible for 90% of adult malignancy.

Acute bleed: bleeding that begins and worsen quickly; not chronic.

Adenocarcinoma of the colon: the most common type of colon cancer.

Adenoma: a precancerous tumor.

Adenomatous polyposis coli (ACP): the gene associated with the hereditary disease Familial Adenomatous Polyposis.

Adenomatous polyps: a polyp that has transformed to a pre-cancerous state

Adjuvant therapy: treatment given after the primary treatment to increase the chances of a cure. Adjuvant therapy may include chemotherapy, radiation therapy, hormone therapy, or biological therapy.

Alternative therapies: unconventional cancer therapies offered as replacement to standard modalities of chemotherapy and radiation; not recognized by medical establishment or insurers; often untested but supported by personal anecdote.

Amino acids: specific types of chemical compounds that are the building blocks of proteins.

Aorta: The main artery of the body.

Anal sphincter: the muscular valve separating the rectum and anus that controls the exit of solid waste (feces).

Anastomosis: a procedure to connect healthy sections of tubular structures in the body after the diseased portion has been surgically removed.

Anemia: a condition characterized by a decreased amount of red blood cells. (Anemic=Adj.)

Aneuploid: having an abnormal number of sets of chromosomes; for example, tetraploid means having two paired sets of chromosomes, which is twice as many as normal; aneuploid cancer cells tend not to respond as well to therapy; aneuploidy refers to the state of being aneuploid. *See also* **diploid** *and* **ploidy**.

Anterior: anatomic term referring to plane of the body associated with nose, naval, and knee

Anus: the opening of the rectum to the outside of the body.

Agiogenesis factor: refers to a substance that tumors produce in order to grow new blood vessels.

Amino acids: the chemical building blocks of proteins.

Appendix: a small outporching of the distal ileum.

Ascending colon: the first portion of the large intestines.

Avastin: a targeted systemic therapy also known as a VEGF inhibitor.

Barium enema: a procedure in which a liquid with barium in it is put into the rectum and colon by way of the anus; barium is a silver-white metallic compound that helps to show the image of the lower gastrointestinal tract on an x-ray. *See also* **double contrast barium enema.**

Benign: relatively harmless; not cancerous; not malignant.

Best supportive care: the care concept whereby the cancer patient is managed without directed anti-cancer therapy.

Bevacizumab: *See* **Avastin.**

Bile: a chemical synthesized in the liver and secreted into the small intestine to facilitate the uptake of nutrients from food.

Biological therapy: treatment to stimulate or restore the ability of the immune (defense) system to fight infection and disease; also called immunotherapy.

Biopsy: the removal of a sample of tissue from a particular part of the body in order to check for abnormalities such as cancer; removed tissue is typically examined microscopically by a pathologist in order to make a precise diagnosis of the patient's condition.

Bone scan: a technique that is more sensitive than conventional x-rays, it uses a radio-labeled agent to identify abnormal or cancerous growths within or attached to bone; in the case of colon cancer, a bone scan is used to identify bone metastases; metastases appear as "hot spots" on the film; however, the absence of hot spots does not prove the absence of tiny metastases.

Bowel: the long, tube-shaped organ in the abdomen that completes the process of digestion; there is both a small and a large bowel; also called the intestine.

Bowel continence: the ability to control the exit of fecal waste from the body.

Bowel incontinence: the inability to control the exit of fecal waste from the body.

Bowel movements: the passage of fecal waste out of the body.

Brush biopsy: a biopsy facilitated by moving a brush across the surface of a suspicious lesion.

Capecitabine: an oral chemotherapy base of 5FU.

Carbohydrate: a sugar molecule; carbohydrates can be small and simple (for example, glucose) or they can be large and complex (for example, polysaccharides such as starch, chitin, or cellulose).

Cancer: a term for the diseases in which abnormal cells divide without control; cancer cells can invade surrounding tissue and spread to other parts of the body through the bloodstream and lymphatic system.

Cancer prevention: the active process of decreasing cancer incidence in a population.

Cancer relapse: cancer recurrence.

Carcino embryonic antigen (CEA): *See* **CEA**.

Carcinogen: a chemical or agent that promotes cellular transformation to cancer.

Carcinogenesis: the sequential genetic and molecular changes that are responsible for cellular transformations into cancer.

Carcinoma: a form of cancer that originates in organ tissues as a result of transformation of the epithelial cells.

Carcinoma in situ: cancer that involves only cells in the tissue in which it began and that has not spread to nearby tissues.

Caudad: an anatomic term indicating a direction toward the feet.

CEA: carcinoembryonic antigen; a substance that is sometimes found in an increased amount in the blood of people who have certain cancers, other diseases, or who smoke. It is used as a tumor marker for colorectal cancer.

CEA assay: a laboratory test to measure the level of carcinoembryonic antigen (CEA).

Cecum: the anatomic transition area between the small and large intestines.

Cephalad: an anatomic term indicating a direction toward the head.

Cetuximab: *See* **Erbitux**.

Chemoprevention: the use of a pharmaceutical or other substance to prevent the development of cancer.

Chemotherapy: the use of pharmaceuticals or other chemicals to kill cancer cells; in many cases, chemotherapeutic agents kill not only cancer cells but also other cells in the body, making such agents potentially very dangerous.

Chromosome: a thread-like linear strand of DNA and associated proteins in the nucleus of cells that carries the genes and functions in the transmission of hereditary information.

Chronic bleed: slow insidious bleeding for which the body compensates.

CIS: *See* **carcinoma in situ**.

Clean margin: *See* **margin**.

Clinical trial: a carefully planned experiment to evaluate a treatment or a medication (often a new pharmaceutical) for an unproven use; phase 1 trials are very preliminary, short-term trials involving a few patients designed to evaluate safety; phase 2 trials may involve 20 to 50 patients and are designed to estimate the most active dose of a new drug and evaluate efficiency; phase 3 trials involve many patients and compare a new therapy against the current standard or best available therapy to evaluate superiority.

Close margin: *See* **margin**.

Colectomy: an operation to remove all or part of the colon; when only part of the colon is removed; it is called a partial colectomy. In an open colectomy, one long incision is made in the wall of the abdomen and doctors can see the colon directly; in a laparoscopic-assisted colectomy, several small incisions are made and a thin, lighted tube attached to a video camera is inserted through one opening to guide the surgery, while surgical instruments are inserted through the other openings to perform the surgery.

Collumnators: the device within a linear accelerator that regulates the dose of radiation exposure.

Colon: the longest part of the large intestine; the colon removes water and some nutrients and electrolytes from partially digested food. The remaining material, solid waste called stool, moves through the colon to the rectum and leaves the body through the anus.

Colonoscope: a thin, lighted tube used to examine the inside of the colon.

Colonoscopy: an examination of the inside of the colon using a thin, lighted tube, called a colonoscope, inserted into the rectum; samples of tissues may be collected for examination under a microscope.

Colostomy: an opening into the colon from the outside of the body; a colostomy provides a new path for waste material to leave the body after part of the colon has been removed.

Complementary therapies: unconventional therapies that can be effectively integrated into standard medical care but are not necessarily endorsed by the medical establishment or proven to improve outcomes by evidence-based criteria.

Complication: an unexpected or unwanted effect of a treatment, pharmaceutical, or other procedure.

Computerized axial tomography (CAT or CT scan): a method of combining images from multiple x-rays under the control of a computer to produce cross-sectional or three-dimensional pictures of the internal organs that can be used to identify abnormalities; used for evaluating metastases of the lymph nodes or more distant soft tissue sites.

Congenital mutations: gene alterations that develop in utero.

Constipation: a condition in which stool becomes hard, dry, and difficult to pass, and bowel movements don't happen very often; other symptoms may include painful bowel movements and feeling bloated, uncomfortable, and sluggish.

Crypt cells: mucosal cells of the colon responsible for water reclamation.

CT scan: *See* **computerized axil tomography scan**.

Defecation: the passage of fecal waste.

De-novo acquired mutations: a newly acquired mutation that confers risk to future generations.

Descending colon: the third portion of the colon.

Diagnosis: the evaluation of signs, symptoms, and selected test results by a physician to determine the physical and biological causes of the signs and symptoms and whether or not a specific disease or disorder is involved.

Diarrhea: frequent and watery bowel movements.

Differentiation: (1) the process by which the homogenous cells of the developing embryo change into the 200+ cell types of the human being and the process showing how mature (developed) the cancer cells are in a tumor; (2) differentiated tumor cells resemble normal cells and grow at a slower rate than undifferentiated tumor cells, which lack the structure and function of normal cells and grow more aggressively.

Digested: decomposed food prepared for absorption of nutrients.

Digestive enzymes: chemicals secreted by the upper GI tract organs that facilitate food decomposition.

Digestive system: the organs that take in food and turn it into products that the body can use to stay healthy; waste products the body cannot use leave the body through bowel movements; the digestive system includes the salivary glands, mouth, esophagus, stomach, liver, pancreas, gallbladder, small and large intestines, and rectum.

Digital rectal exam (DRE): an exam to detect rectal cancer; the doctor inserts a lubricated, gloved finger into the rectum and feels for abnormal areas.

Diploid: having one complete set of normally paired chromosomes, that is, a normal amount of DNA; a diploid number of chromosomes would equal 46, and a haploid set would equal 23. *See also* **ploidy**.

Disease-specific survival: the measurement of life-expectancy specific to a disease process.

Distal: an anatomic term indicating a direction toward the end.

DNA: the basic biologically active chemical that defines the physical development and growth of nearly all living organisms; a complex protein that is the carrier of genetic information.

Double contrast barium enema (DCBE): *See* **barium enema**.

Duodenum: the first portion of the small intestine.

Ectoderm: the layer of pre-embryologic cells that gives rise to skin and nerves.

Electromagnetic spectrum: the range of radiant energy that is distinguished by wavelength and includes therapeutic radiation, visible light, radio waves, etc.

Embryo: the human in its earliest stage of intrauterine development.

En-bloc resection: a surgical procedure in which a tumor is removed in its entirely without any disruption of its surface.

Endoderm: the layer of cells in the developing embryo that gives rise to the body's organs.

Endoscopic polypectomy: surgical removal of a polyp via an endoscope.

Enterostomal therapist: a healthcare specialist trained to help patients care for and adjust to their colostomy.

Enzyme: any of a group of chemical substances that are produced by living cells and that cause particular chemical reactions to happen while not being changed themselves.

Epidermal growth factor (EGF): a ligand associated with epithelial tumor cell growth and proliferation.

Epithelial cell: those cells derived from the endoderm and that comprise the organs.

Eribitux: a targeted therapy directed at the EGF receptor.

Esophageal sphincter: the muscular valve that prevents food from re-entering the esophagus once it enters the stomach.

Esophagus: the muscular tube through which food passes from the throat to the stomach.

Estrogen: a sex hormone associated with female secondary sex characteristics.

Estrogen receptor: the docking site on the cell for estrogen. It is a protein that can be measured and quantified.

Excisional biopsy: the removal of an area of diseased tissue in its entirety for submission for pathologic review.

Exploratory laparotomy: the surgical procedure in which the abdominal cavity is opened and directly evaluated for disease process.

External beam radiation therapy: a form of radiation therapy in which the radiation is delivered by a machine directed at the area to be radiated as opposed to radiation given within the target tissue such as brachytherapy.

Familial adenomatous polyposis: FAP. An inherited condition in which numerous polyps (growths that protrude from mucous membranes) form on the inside walls of the colon and rectum. It increases the risk of colorectal cancer. Also called familial polyposis.

Family history: *See* **pedigree.**

Fecal incontinence: *See* **bowel incontinence.**

Fecal occult blood test (FOBT): a test to check for blood in the stool; small samples of stool are placed on specials cards and sent to a doctor or laboratory for testing; blood in the stool may be a sign of colorectal cancer.

Fiber: the parts of fruits and vegetables that cannot be digested; also called bulk or roughage.

Fine-needle aspiration: removal of cellular material from diseased tissue via a needle for submission for pathologic review.

Fluorouracil (5-Fluorouracil, 5FU): *See* **5-Fluorouracil.**

Flow cytometry: a measurement method that determines the fraction of cells that are diploid, tetraploid, aneuploid, etc. (ploidy status), as well as the percent of DNA undergoing synthesis (S-phase).

Fluorescent in situ hybridization: a laboratory technique that can identify specific DNA sequences.

Folfox 4: the acronym for a chemotherapy regimen with 5FU + Oxaliplatin.

Folinic acid: Also called leukovorin, a vitamin that augments 5FU activity.

Forceps biopsy: a pincer device used to obtain tissue for pathologic review.

Fraction: the portion of a fractionated radiation treatment that is delivered in a single session.

Freedom from progression: an outcome measure that identifies the time between a treatment and subsequent re-growth of cancer.

Gall bladder: the organ that stores bile.

Gamma radiation: very short wavelength electromagnetic radiation used for therapeutic radiation.

Gastroenterologist: a doctor who specializes in diagnosing and treating diseases of the digestive system.

Gastrointestinal tract: the stomach and intestines.

Gene: a discrete DNA sequence that codes for a specific protein.

Genetic code: the complete gene sequence of an organism mapped out in its respective DNA code.

Genome: the total genetic content contained in a haploid set of chromosomes in single or multicelled organisms, in a single chromosome in bacteria, or in the DNA or RNA of viruses; an organism's genetic material.

Genomics: the study of genomic instability.

GI tract: the series of organs from mouth to anus through which food travels.

Glandular tissue: epithelial tissue that has the capacity to secrete or absorb.

Haustra: the circular muscle bands of the colon that facilitate peristalsis and give the colon the appearance of segmentation.

Hemoglobin: the substance inside red blood cells that binds to oxygen and carries it from the lungs to the tissues.

Hepatic flexure: the location near the liver where the ascending colon is fixed in position and transitions to the transverse colon.

Hereditary: transmitted from parent to child by information contained in the genes.

Hereditary non-polyposis colon cancer syndrome (HNPCC): an inherited disorder in which affected individuals have a higher than normal chance of developing colorectal cancer and certain other types of cancer, often before the age of 50; also called Lynch syndrome.

Histologic grade: a system that attempts to quantify a pathologist's subjective interpretation of a cell's degree of differentiation.

Homogeneous (homogeneity): uniform; composed of the same element; in reference to a tumor cell population, it means that the cells are of the same clone, in contrast to a mixed-cell population that would exhibit heterogeneity or be heterogeneous.

Hormones: biologically active chemicals that are secreted by one organ and that then travel through the circulation, where they exert effort elsewhere.

Hormone therapy: the use of hormones, hormone analogues, and certain surgical techniques to treat disease either on their own or in combination with other hormones or in combination with other methods of treatment.

Hyperplasia: the earliest change of duct cell growth, characterized by orderly overgrowth.

Hyperplastic polyps: mucosal epithelial overgrown localized to a growth.

Ileostomy: an opening created by a surgeon into the ileum (part of the small intestine) from the outside of the body; an ileostomy provides a new path for waste material to leave the body after part of the intestine has been removed.

Ileum: the third or terminal portion of the small intestines.

Immune system: The complex group of organs and cells that defends the body against infection or disease.

Immune system: the biological system that protects a person or animal from the effects of foreign materials such as bacteria, viruses, and other things that might make that person or animal sick.

Imaging: a radiology technique or method allowing a physician to see something that would not be visible to the unaided eye.

Injection: the use of a syringe and needle to push fluids or drugs into the body; often called a shot.

Intestine: the long, tube-shaped organ in the abdomen that completes the process of digestion; there is both a large intestine and small intestine; also called the bowel.

Incisional biopsy: surgical removal of a piece of diseased tissue for submission for pathologic review.

Infiltrating tumor: *See* **invasive colonic adenocarcinoma**.

Informed consent: permission to proceed given by a patient after being fully informed of the purposes and potential consequences of a medical procedure.

Interventional Radiology: A specialized radiology department that performs surgical procedures requiring imaging guidance.

Intraperitoneal: within the peritoneal cavity (the area that contains the abdominal organs).

Invasive colonic adenocarcinoma: the most advanced local presentation of a colorectal cancer where it no longer respects the mucosa as a boundary but invades or infiltrates submucosasal tissues, blood, and lymphatic channels.

Irinotecan: a chemotherapy drug.

Jejunum: the second portion of the small intestines.

Juvenile polyps: a type of benign polyp.

Laparoscopy: the procedure in which the intra-abdominal organs are evaluated though the laparoscope.

LAR: See **Lower anterior resection**.

Large bowel: another term for colon.

Iron deficiency: inadequate storage iron often presenting as anemia.

Large intestine: the long, tube-like organ that is connected to the small intestine at one end and the anus at the other end; the large intestine has four parts (cecum, colon, rectum, and anus canal); partly digested food moves through the cecum into the colon, where water and some nutrients and electrolytes are removed; the remaining material, solid waste called stool, moves through the colon, is stored in the rectum, and leaves the body through the anal canal and anus.

Lateral: an anatomic reference to those structures away from the midline.

Left hemicolectomy: a surgical procedure that removes the left or descending colon.

Levcovorin: *See* **folinic acid**.

Levamisole: an immuomadulating drug once thought to be active in colon cancer.

Ligand: a circulating chemical that can interact with a cell via a receptor triggering intracellulous events.

Linear accelerator: the machine that delivers therapeutic external radiation.

Liver: a large organ located in the upper abdomen; the liver cleanses the blood and aids in digestion by secreting bile.

Local cancer: an invasive malignant cancer confined entirely to the organ where the cancer began.

Localized: restricted to a well-defined area.

Local recurrence: a relapse of cancer.

Lower anterior resection: the surgical procedure that removes the rectum but preserves the anal sphincter.

Local therapy: Treatment that affects only a tumor and the area close to it.

Lower GI series: a series of x-rays of the colon and rectum that is taken after the patient is given a barium enema.

Lower GI tract: a common term for the colon and rectum.

Lymph: the clear fluid in which all of the cells in the body are constantly bathed; carries cells that help fight infection; also called lymphatic fluid.

Lymphatic system: the tissue and organs that produce, store, and carry cells that fight infection; includes bone marrow, spleen, thymus, lymph nodes, and channels that carry lymph fluid.

Lymph nodes: the small glands that occur throughout the body and that filter the clear fluid known as lymph or lymphatic fluid; lymph nodes filter out bacteria and other toxins, as well as cancer cells.

Magnetic resonance: absorption of specific frequencies of radio and microwave radiation by atoms placed in a strong magnetic field.

Magnetic resonance imaging: the use of magnetic resonance with atoms in body tissues to produce distinct cross-sectional and even three-dimensional images of internal organs.

Malignancy: a growth or tumor composed of cancerous cells.

Malignant: cancerous; tending to become progressively worse and to result in death; having the invasive and metastatic (spreading) properties of cancer.

Margin: normally used to mean the surgical margin, which is the outer edge of the tissue removed during surgery; if the surgical margin shows no sign of cancer, then it is a negative or clear margin; if the margin is equivocal then it is a close margin; if the margin has definite cancer, then it is a positive, dirty, or involved margin.

Medial: an anatomic term indicating a direction toward the midline.

Medical oncologist: an oncologist primarily trained in the use of medicines (rather than surgery) to treat cancer.

Melena: bowel movement of decomposed blood.

Mesentery: the connective tissue that is affixed to the first three segments of the colon.

Mesoderm: the middle cellular layer of the developing embryo that gives rise to blood, muscle, and bone.

Meta-analysis: a statistical method that combines many related but not identical clinical trial outcomes to assess meaningful trends in patient treatment.

Metastasis (plural is metastases): a secondary tumor formed as a result of a cancer cell or cells from the primary tumor site traveling through the blood circulation to a new site and then growing there.

Metastasize: spread of a malignant tumor to other parts of the body.

Metastatic: having the characteristics of a secondary cancer.

Metastatic therapy: the treatment of proven and measurable metastases.

Microarray testing: the study of genes and proteins likely to predict cancer risk.

Microcytic anemia: the category of anemia to which iron deficiency belongs characterized by small red blood cells.

Micrometastases: metastases that is too small to be measured by conventional testing.

Microsatellite instability (MSI): a genetic abnormality associated with colon cancer.

Mismatch Repair Gene (MMR) Mutation: mutation associated with HNPCC.

Morbidity: unhealthy consequences and complications resulting from treatment.

Mucosa: the inside layer or lining of the gastrointestinal organs.

Muscularis: the middle or muscular layer of gastrointestinal organs.

Mutation: a defect in a DNA nucleoside base sequence that can lead to altered gene expression.

National Surgical Adjuvant Breast and Bowel Project (NSABP): a prominent cooperative group of cancer researchers that conducts clinical trials in breast and colorectal cancers.

Neoadjuvant: the use of a different kind of therapy before the use of what is considered a more definitive therapy (e.g., the use of neoadjuvant chemo radiation therapy before surgery for rectal cancer); neoadjuvant is contrasted to adjuvant, which relates to the use of another therapy after the more definitive therapy.

Neoplasm: another term for cancer. Latin for "new growth."

Neoplasia: the growth of cells under conditions that would tend to prevent the development of normal tissue (e.g., a cancer).

Nuclear grade: a system that attempts to quantify a pathologist's subjective interpretation of a cell's nuclear abnormality.

Nucleoside bases: the four characters representing the chemical code for DNA.

Nutrient: a chemical compound (such as protein, fat, carbohydrate, vitamins, or minerals) that makes up food. These compounds are used by the body to function and grow.

Obstruction: a blockage; term usually used in reference to the flow of fecal waste.

Occult blood loss: unobserved bleeding in the gastrointestinal tract often found as a result of iron deficiency.

Oligometases: isolated metastases, usually three or less, and usually restricted to a single site (e.g., liver or lung).

Oncologist: a physician who specializes in the treatment of various types of cancer.

Oncology: the branch of medical science dealing with tumors.

Organ: a group of tissues that work in concert to carry out a specific set of functions (e.g., the heart or the lungs or the breast).

Ostomy: an operation to create an opening from an area inside the body to the outside. *See* **colostomy**.

Overall survival: an outcome measure that references years of life after a cancer treatment.

Oxaliplatin: a chemotherapy drug.

Palliative: designed to relieve a particular problem without necessarily solving it; for example, palliative therapy is given in order to relieve symptoms and improve quality of life but does not cure the patient.

Palliative therapy: treatment given to relieve the symptoms and reduce the sufferings caused by cancer and other life-threatening diseases; palliative cancer therapies are given together with other cancer treatments, from the time of diagnosis, through treatment, survivorship, recurrent, or advanced disease, and at the end of life.

Palpable: capable of being felt during a physical examination by an experienced physician.

Partial response: a 50% or greater decline in parameters that are being used to measure anticancer activity; parameters include abnormalities found using physical exams and laboratory and radiologic studies.

Pedigree: a term used to reference an individual's genetic lineage.

Pathologist: a physician who specializes in the examination of tissue and blood samples to help decide what diseases are present and therefore how they should be treated.

Pedunculated: a mushroom-like growth.

Perforation: a rupture or hole through the wall of the colon.

Perineal cavity: *See* **pelvic cavity**.

Perineum: the area of skin surrounding the genitals and anus.

Peritoneal cavity: *See* **abdominal cavity**.

Peristatsis: the forward propulsion of digested food through the gastrointestinaltract.

Pelvis: the bones of the lower trunk.

Pelvic cavity: the cavity outlined by the pelvic bones and sacrum.

Peritoneum: the tissue that lines the abdominal wall and covers most of the organs in the abdomen.

PET Scan: *See* **positron emission tomography**.

Phase 1 clinical trial: a clinical trial that addresses toxicity.

Phase 2 clinical trial: a clinical trial that addresses efficiency.

Phase 3 clinical trial: a clinical trial that compares an efficacious agent or procedure with acceptable toxicity to a current standard of care.

Placebo: a form of safe but nonactive treatment frequently used as a basis for comparison with pharmaceuticals in research studies.

Plasma: the viscous fluid of blood where the blood cells are suspended.

Platelet: a blood cell involved in blood clotting.

Ploidy: a term used to describe the number or sets of chromosomes in a cell. *See* **diploid** and **aneuploid**.

Polyp: a mass of tissue that develops on the inside wall of a hollow organ such as the colon.

Polypectomy: surgery to remove a polyp.

Port: an implanted venous access device.

Positron Emission Tomography (PET scan): a scan using a radioactive isotope that is taken up by tumor tissue showing that the tumor is functional.

Posterior: an anatomic term referencing the plane of the body comprised of heel, buttocks and occiput.

Primary systemic: *See* **neoadjuvant.**

Prognosis: the likely outcome or course of a disease; the chance of recovery or recurrence.

Prognostic criteria: features of a cancer that fall outside traditional staging criteria but nonetheless are predictive of outcome.

Progression: continuing growth or regrowth of the cancer.

Prophylactic: preventative.

Protein: one of three major chemical classes found in living matter along with fats and carbohydrates; the machines of cells.

Proteinomics: the study of proteins resulting from genomic instability.

Protocol: a precise set of methods by which a research study is to be carried out.

Proximal: an anatomic term indicating a direction toward the origin (e.g., in GI reference, the mouth).

PSA (prostate specific antigen): a chemical found in the normal prostate gland that may elevate in the blood when the gland undergoes cancer transformation.

Pyloric sphincter: a muscular valve that controls the exit of stomach contents.

Quality of life: The overall enjoyment of life. Many clinical trials assess the effects of cancer and its treatment on the quality of life. Theses studies measure aspects of an individual's sense of well-being and ability to carry out various activities.

Radiant energy: *See* **electromagnetic spectrum**.

Radiation oncologist: a physician who has received special training regarding the treatment of cancers with different types of radiation.

Radiation therapy: the use of x-rays and other forms of radiation to destroy malignant cells and tissue.

Radiotherapy: *See* **radiation therapy**.

Radiofrequency ablation: also referred to as RFA; a procedure where a microwave-emitting probe is imbedded into a tumor and destroys it.

Randomized: a feature of clinical trials whereby participants are assigned to different treatments to remove investigator bias.

Receptor: a docking site that interacts with a ligand (e.g., estrogen); receptors may be on the cell membrane or within the cell cytoplasm or nucleus; estrogen receptors are examples; all cells have multiple receptors.

Recurrence: a relapse or re-growth of cancer; the reappearance of disease; this can be manifested clinically as findings on the physical examination or as a laboratory recurrence or as an imaging finding.

Rectum: the last 6 to 8 inches of the large intestine; the rectum stores solid waste until it leaves the body through the anus.

Recurrent cancer: cancer that has returned after a period of time during which the cancer could not be detected; the cancer may come back to the same place as the original (primary) tumor or to another place in the body; also called recurrence.

Red blood cell (RBC): one of three blood cell classes along with white blood cells and platelets; responsible for oxygen transport throughout the body; also called an erythrocyte.

Regression: the real or apparent disappearance of some or all of the signs and symptoms of cancer; the period (temporary or permanent) during which a disease remains under control, without progressing; even complete remission does not necessarily indicate cure.

Relapse-free progression: *See* **freedom from progression**.

Remission: the measurable repression or shrinkage of a cancer; may be qualified as partial, complete, clinical, etc.

Resection: surgical removal.

Response: a decrease in disease that occurs because of treatment; divided into complete response (remission), partial response (remission), clinical response (by exam), radiologic response (by imaging), pathologic response (by microscopic review), etc.

Ribosome: the organelle within a cell's cytoplasm responsible for protein synthesis.

Right hemicolectomy: the surgical procedure for the removal of the ascending colon.

Risk: the chance or probability that a particular event will or will not happen.

RNA: the genetic material that transmits the DNA message from the nucleus to the cytoplasm.

Salvage: a procedure intended to "rescue" a patient after the failure of a prior treatment.

Screening: evaluating populations of people to diagnose disease early.

Segmental colectomy: the surgical removal of a small diseased segment of the colon.

Sensitivity: the probability that a diagnostic test can correctly identify the presence of a particular disease assuming the proper conduct of the test; specifically, the number of true positive results divided by the sum of the true positive results and the false negative results. *See* **specificity**.

Serosa: the outer or protective layer of the gastrointestinal organs.

Sessile: a flat growth.

Side effect: a reaction to medication or treatment (most commonly used to mean an unnecessary or undesirable effect).

Sigmoid colectomy: the surgical procedure to remove the sigmoid colon.

Sigmoid colon: the fourth segment of the colon.

Sigmoidoscope: a thin, lighted tube used to view the inside of the colon.

Sigmoidoscopy: inspection of the rectum and lower colon using a thin, lighted tube called a sigmoidoscope; samples of tissue or cells may be collected for examination under a microscope; also called protosigmoidoscopy.

Small intestine: the part of the digestive tract that is located between the stomach and the large intestine.

Specificity: the probability that a diagnostic test can correctly identify the absence of a particular disease, assuming the proper conduct of the test; specifically, the number of true negative results divided by the sum of the true negative results and the false positive results; a method that detects 95% of true cancer cases is highly sensitive, but if it also falsely indicates that 40% of those who do not have cancer do have cancer, then its specificity is 60% (rather poor).

S-phase: *See* **flow cytometry**.

Splenic flexure: the anatomic location where the colon is fixed and transitions from transverse to descending segments.

Squamous cell carcinoma: squamous epithelial cells that have undergone cancerous transformation.

Stage: the extent of a cancer in the body; staging is usually based on the size of the tumor, whether or not lymph nodes contain cancer, and whether or not the cancer has spread from the original site to other parts of the body.

Stage 0 colorectal cancer: cancer is found in the innermost lining of the colon and/or rectum only; also called carcinoma in situ.

Stage I colorectal cancer: cancer has spread beyond the innermost lining of the colon and/or rectum to the second and third layers and involves the inside wall of the colon and/or rectum, but it has not spread to the outer wall or outside the colon and/or rectum.

Stage II colorectal cancer: cancer has spread outside the colon and/or rectum to nearby tissue, but it has not gone into the lymph nodes; also called Dukes' B colorectal cancer.

Stage III colorectal cancer: tumor cells have spread to organs and lymph nodes near the colon/rectum; also called Dukes' C colorectal cancer.

Stage IV colorectal cancer: cancer may have spread to nearby lymph nodes and has spread to other parts of the body.

Staging: performing exams and tests to learn the extent of the cancer within the body, especially whether or not the disease has spread from the original site to other parts of the body; it is important to know the stage of the disease in order to plan the best treatment.

Standard therapy: in medicine, treatment that experts agree is appropriate, accepted, and widely used; healthcare providers are obligated to provide patients with standard therapy; also called standard of care or best practice.

Stoma: a surgically created opening into the body from the outside.

Stomach: an organ that is part of the digestive system; it helps in the digestion of food by mixing it with digestive juices and churning it into a thin liquid.

Stool: The solid waste matter discharged in a bowel movement; feces.

Support drugs: medications that have no inherent anticancer activity but improve the tolerance and safety of standard treatment.

Surgery: a procedure to remove or repair a part of the body or to find out whether or not disease is present; an operation.

Survival: length of life after a diagnosis.

Symptom: a feeling, sensation, or experience associated with or resulting from a physical or mental disorder and noticeable by the patient.

Systemic: throughout the whole body; affecting the entire body.

Systemic chemotherapy: treatment with anticancer drugs that travel through the blood to cells all over the body.

Systemic therapy: a therapy designed to be effective throughout the entire body.

Targeted therapy: therapies designed to target unique molecular structures.

Therapy: the treatment of disease or disability.

Time to progression: an outcome measure indicating the duration of remission or response to a cancer intervention.

Tissue: a group or layer of cells that perform specific functions.

TNM staging system: a system for quantifying the extent of malignancy by numerically "grading" the size and extent of the primary tumor, the degree of involvement of lymph nodes, and the presence or absence of distant spread (metastases).

Total colectomy: the surgical removal of the entire colon.

Transverse colon: the second segment of the colon.

Treatment: administration of remedies to a patient for a disease.

Treatment surveillance: monitoring of the cancer patient while on an active therapy.

Tubular polyps: benign polyps.

Tubulovillous: a mixed polyp with more aggressive behavior.

Tumor: an excessive growth of cells caused by uncontrolled and disorderly cell replacement; an abnormal tissue growth that can be either benign or malignant. *See* **benign** and **malignant**.

Ulcerative colitis: Chronic inflammation of the colon that produces ulcers in its lining. This condition is marked by abdominal pain, cramps, and loose discharges of pus, blood, and mucus from the bowel.

Ultrasound: sound waves at a particular frequency (far beyond the hearing range) whose echoes bouncing off tissue can be used to image internal organs (e.g., a baby in the womb).

Ultrasonography: a test in which sound waves (ultrasound) are bounced off tissues and the echoes are converted into a picture (sonogram).

Upper GI tract: the organs of the gastrointestinal tract proximal to the colon.

Vascular endothelial growth factor (VEGF): a molecule associated with promoting new blood vessel growth.

Vena Cava: The main vein of the body.

Villous polyps: flat polyps that are often pre-malignant.

Virtual colonoscopy: a method under study to examine the colon by taking a series of x-rays (called a CT scan) and using a high-powered computer to reconstruct 2-D and 3-D pictures of the interior surfaces of the colon; the pictures can be saved, manipulated to better viewing angles, and reviewed after the procedure, even years later; also called computed tomography colography.

Vitamin: a key nutrient that the body needs in small amounts to grow and stay strong. Examples are vitamins A, C, and E.

Wavelengths: *See* **electromagnetic spectrum.**

White blood cell (WBC): refers to a blood cell that does not contain hemoglobin; white blood cells include lymphocytes, neutrophils, eosinophils, macrophages, and mast cells. These cells are made by bone marrow and help the body fight infection and other diseases.

Index

STAGING 53, 73
STANDARD OF CARE 66
STOMACH 6
STOOL xv
surgery xvi
surgical pathology 53
SURVIVAL 89
SUTURE LINE 98
SYMPTOM 23
SYSTEMIC 53
systemic theory of cancer, 60
SYSTEMIC THERAPY 72
Systemic Therapy 78

T

T3 xvii
Tamoxifen 107
TARGETED THERAPY 60, 80
targeted therapy 84
television 67
testosterone 82
Therapeutic radiation 66
The Polyp 26
Three-dimensional imaging 60
TIME TO PROGRESSION 89
TISSUES 5
tissues that comprise the colon and rec-
   tum 11
TNM classification 74
TNM STAGING SYSTEM 73
TOTAL COLECTOMY 58
Total Colectomy 65
Total Proctocolectomy 65
toxicity of chemotherapy 80
translate the human genome 81
transverse colon 10, 63
treatment of metastatic colorectal cancer
   82

treatment options 54
TUBULAR 28
TUBULOVILLOUS 28
TUMOR xv,xvii, 51, 54, 63

U

ULTRASOUND xvii
UPPER GI TRACT 7
ureters 11
urinary tract 31

V

VASCULAR ENDOTHELIAL
   GROWTH FACTOR 82
VECTIBIX 83
Vectibix 87
VEGF 82. See also VASCULAR ENDO-
   THELIAL
      GROWTH FACTOR.
vena cava 11
VILLOUS 28
   adenomas 28
VIRTUAL COLONOSCOPY 30, 36
VITAMIN 86

W

WAVELENGTHS 67
WHITE BLOOD CELLS 56
www.adjuvantonline.com 90

X

x-rays 51
XELODA 87